T0091926

MACRONEURAL THEORIES IN COGNITIVE NEUROSCIENCE

In this book, William R. Uttal continues his analysis and critique of theories of mind. He considers theories that are based on macroneural responses (such as those obtained from fMRI) that represent the averaged or cumulative responses of many neurons. The analysis is carried out with special emphasis on the logical and conceptual difficulties in developing a theory but with special attention to some of the current attempts to go from these cumulative responses to explanations of the grand question of how the mind is generated by the brain. While acknowledging the importance of these macroneural techniques in the study of the anatomy and physiology of the brain, Uttal concludes that this macroneural approach is not likely to produce a valid neural theory of cognition because the critical information—the states of the individual neurons involved in brain activity becoming mental activity—is actually lost in the process of summation. Controversial topics are considered in detail including discussions of empirical, logical, and technological barriers to theory building in cognitive neuroscience.

William R. Uttal is Professor Emeritus (Engineering) at Arizona State University and Professor Emeritus (Psychology) at the University of Michigan. He was one of the pioneering researchers in cognitive neuroscience and is the author of numerous books and over 140 scholarly articles.

Books by William R. Uttal

- *Real Time Computers: Techniques and Applications in the Psychological Sciences*
- *Generative Computer Assisted Instruction* (with Miriam Rogers, Ramelle Hieronymus, and Timothy Pasich)
- *Sensory Coding: Selected Readings* (Editor)
- *The Psychobiology of Sensory Coding*
- *Cellular Neurophysiology and Integration: An Interpretive Introduction*
- *An Autocorrelation Theory of Form Detection*
- *The Psychobiology of Mind*
- *A Taxonomy of Visual Processes*
- *Visual Form Detection in 3-Dimensional Space*
- *Foundations of Psychobiology* (with Daniel N. Robinson)
- *The Detection of Nonplanar Surfaces in Visual Space*
- *The Perception of Dotted Forms*
- *On Seeing Forms*
- *The Swimmer: An Integrated Computational Model of a Perceptual-Motor System* (with Gary Bradshaw, Sriram Dayanand, Robb Lovell, Thomas Shepherd, Ramakrishna Kakarala, Kurt Skifsted, and Greg Tupper)
- *Toward A New Behaviorism: The Case against Perceptual Reductionism*
- *Computational Modeling of Vision: The Role of Combination* (with Ramakrishna Kakarala, Sriram Dayanand, Thomas Shepherd, Jaggi Kalki, Charles Lunskis Jr., and Ning Liu)
- *The War between Mentalism and Behaviorism: On the Accessibility of Mental Processes*
- *The New Phrenology: On the Localization of Cognitive Processes in the Brain*
- *A Behaviorist Looks at Form Recognition*
- *Psychomythics: Sources of Artifacts and Misrepresentations in Scientific Cognitive Neuroscience*
- *Dualism: The Original Sin of Cognitivism*
- *Neural Theories of Mind: Why the Mind-Brain Problem May Never Be Solved*
- *Human Factors in the Courtroom: Mythology versus Science*
- *The Immeasurable Mind: The Real Science of Psychology*
- *Time, Space, and Number in Physics and Psychology*
- *Distributed Neural Systems: Beyond the New Phrenology*
- *Neuroscience in the Courtroom: What Every Lawyer Should Know about the Mind and the Brain*
- *Mind and Brain: A Critical Appraisal of Cognitive Neuroscience*
- *Reliability in Cognitive Neuroscience: A Meta-Meta-Analysis*
- *The Case against Macroneural Theories of the Mind*
- *Macroneural Theories in Cognitive Neuroscience*

MACRONEURAL THEORIES IN COGNITIVE NEUROSCIENCE

William R. Uttal

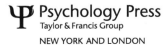

Psychology Press
Taylor & Francis Group
NEW YORK AND LONDON

First published 2016
by Psychology Press
711 Third Avenue, New York, NY 10017

and by Psychology Press
27 Church Road, Hove, East Sussex BN3 2FA

Psychology Press is an imprint of the Taylor & Francis Group, an informa business

© 2016 Taylor & Francis

The right of William R. Uttal to be identified as author of this work has been asserted by him in accordance with sections 77 and 78 of the Copyright, Designs and Patents Act 1988.

All rights reserved. No part of this book may be reprinted or reproduced or utilised in any form or by any electronic, mechanical, or other means, now known or hereafter invented, including photocopying and recording, or in any information storage or retrieval system, without permission in writing from the publishers.

Trademark notice: Product or corporate names may be trademarks or registered trademarks, and are used only for identification and explanation without intent to infringe.

Library of Congress Cataloging-in-Publication Data
A catalog record has been requested for this book

ISBN: 978-1-138-88746-6 (hbk)
ISBN: 978-1-138-88747-3 (pbk)
ISBN: 978-1-315-67895-5 (ebk)

Typeset in Bembo
by Apex CoVantage, LLC

Printed and bound in the United States of America by Publishers Graphics, LLC on sustainably sourced paper.

The relationship between brain and cognition is still only poorly understood. Great progress notwithstanding, neuroscience still cannot answer the "big questions" about mind and intelligence.

(Sporns, 2011, p. 179)

Exercising the right of occasional suppression and slight modification, it is truly absurd to see how plastic a limited number of observations become, in the hands of men with preconceived ideas.

(Galton, 1863, cited in Stigler, 1986, p. 267)

If psychological states are constructed, emergent phenomena, then they will not reveal their more primitive elements, any more than a loaf of bread reveals all the ingredients that constitute it.

(Barrett, 2011, p. 124)

To be brutally honest, scientists do not yet have even the remotest idea of how visual experiences—or indeed any other kind of experiences—arise from physical events in the brain.

(Palmer, 1999, p. 618)

The problem of consciousness is completely intractable. We will never understand consciousness in the deeply satisfying way we've come to expect from our sciences.

(Dietrich & Hardcastle, 2005, cited in Rakover, 2011, p. 18)

A review of the neuroimaging literature suggests that selective association between mental processes and brain structures is currently impossible to find.

(Poldrack, 2010, p. 754)

FOR MITCHAN

CONTENTS

PREFACE

The ultimate goal of cognitive neuroscience is to explain how brain activity produces mental activity. In other words, it is to provide an answer to the age-old mind-body problem, now particularized as the mind-brain problem. Without attaching too much hyperbole to the discussion, it is fair to say that we are asking what may be considered to be the preeminent conundrum of human intellectual history—how does the material brain create the intangible sense of conscious awareness shared by humans and provide for the adaptive cognitive processes that guide our experiences and our behavior? In its extreme complexity, this "problem" crosses over a vast range of intellectual and scientific disciplines including theology, philosophy, mathematics, statistics, and biology, as well as certain fields of psychology.

The answers to this awe-inspiring question have ranged from dualistic concepts asserting that the mental and neural domains were distinctly different kinds of "reality" to those arguing that mind is simply an irrelevant byproduct or epiphenomenon of neuronal activity to modern monist, physicalist, and neuroreductionist identity theories. However, the basic idea guiding current scientific thinking is that whatever mind is, it is nothing more (or less) than an outcome, product, or activity of the material nervous system. Thus, it has been argued that to understand the mind requires that we understand the brain. Indeed, some philosophers even have argued that the definitions and methods of psychology are only temporary substitutes for the ultimate neurophysiological explanations of mind and behavior; neurophysiology, they argued (e.g., Churchland, 1981), will ultimately replace psychological languages, descriptions, theories, and explanations. Obviously, we are nowhere near such an "eliminative" explanation, but the point is made "in principle." In practice, however, such eliminative solutions are at best the hope of some distant future.

Unfortunately, the problem of reducing psychological constructs to neuro-physiological mechanisms has turned out to be far more complex and difficult than originally anticipated. Even the newest and most powerful techniques to study brain anatomy, physiology, and cognitive processes hardly have begun to unravel the "world knot"—the expression of the mind-brain problem attributed to Arthur Schopenhauer (1788–1860). We now know that, beyond its importance, the problem is exceedingly complex. Not only is the brain an intricate network of idiosyncratically interconnected neurons, but also cognition is inadequately defined by such words as "mind," "thinking," "consciousness," and a host of other terms used by psychologists.

This book is concerned with a special aspect of modern cognitive neuroscience theory—the linkage of the findings obtained with macroscopic responses of the brain to human thought processes. It is a sequel to my earlier work *Neural Theories of Mind* (Uttal, 2005), in which I asked similar questions for electric fields, single cells, and neural networks. The answer to which I have arrived is that, for the time being at least, there is no theoretical pathway to answering this question with brain imaging techniques. Although I plan to be as unbiased as possible and present to the extent possible both sides of the question, I must acknowledge that I have concluded that an overarching mind-brain theory is no more likely to arise from any current conceived macroneural approach.

This book is aimed at exploring the role of current macroneural theory in cognitive neuroscience and making the case for its impenetrability. To understand how we might contribute to this discussion, it is necessary to consider what a theory is in general as well as in the particular context of cognitive neuroscience. Over the years, I have explored questions such as the following:

1. What are the properties of a robust theory relating mind and brain?
2. What kinds of mind-brain theories exist?
3. What is an acceptable theory at the macroneural level of brain images?
4. What assumptions have to be made in formulating a modern theory?
5. What are the conditions of necessity and sufficiency that make a theory or law acceptable?
6. Can neural data inform cognitive theory?
7. Can cognitive data inform neural theory?
8. How do description and explanation differ?
9. What is the relation between simulation models to the processes they imitate?
10. How can analogies mislead us into assuming that processes drawn from the psychological and neurophysiological levels are homologous rather than just analogous, coincidental, or correlative?
11. What kind of a balance can be established between achievable pragmatic concerns (medical practice) and what may be logically unachievable biopsychological theories?
12. Which so-called "theories" are only superficial restatements of a priori postulates, intuitions, experimental results, or anecdotal observations?

13. Finally, for cognitive neuroscience, the big question is: Are the data of cognitive neuroscience sufficiently objective, regular, reliable, robust, and far reaching so that a comprehensive theory of mind-brain relations can be constructed from them? Can we look forward to theories that are as well structured, axiomatic, and deductive as are those found, for example, in physics? In other words, are the barriers to developing reductive theories to bridge between the mental and the neurophysiological tractable or intractable?

Obviously, not all of these questions can be resolved within the pages of a single book. Furthermore, it may turn out that some of these questions (e.g., the level of instantiation) may not be answerable in a rigorous fashion; answers being denied by virtue of their complexity or other empirical barriers. However, it seems likely that at least a continuing effort to explore the parameters of what an overarching theory should be like might begin to provide at least a glimmering of answers to some of the questions in this list.

A major issue confronting the theoretician and the experimentalist is the level at which the problem is attacked—the macroneural or the microneuronal. Each has its own difficulties. The macroneural approach is complicated by the cumulative nature of their findings and, thus, the loss of detailed information about the activity of individual neurons. The microneuronal approach, on the other hand, is complicated by the sheer numerousness of the idiosyncratically involved components underlying cognitive activity and their complex interactions. Given these difficulties, there remains a great deal of uncertainty and controversy about what the actual nature of the mind-brain relation is. When interrogated, however, I think that most cognitive neuroscientists would accept the Hebbian (Hebb, 1949) microneuronal answer to the question of the level at which the "meaningful" neural responses are located in the brain. This widely accepted answer is that it is the information transformation processes collectively carried out by innumerable individual neurons, each of which acts as a part of a heavily and idiosyncratically interconnected network, is most likely to be the source of our thoughts, minds, consciousness, cognitive processes, or whatever term one might wish to use. However, it is also probably true that the complexity and numerousness characterizing the interactions among neurons capable of encoding cognition or consciousness is probably beyond our current ability to study empirically because of simple combinatorial constraints despite current progress on the development of powerful supercomputers. Yet, however plausible and relevant this level of analysis may seem to be, it must be remembered that there is only the beginnings of an empirical foundation for the Hebbian model. No one has ever either manipulated the microdetails of the individual states of the neuronal components of a realistic microneuronal network in a way that controls thoughts. Nor has anyone ever observed the details of how a realistic microneuronal network changes with changes in our mental states. Simulations of the relation between neuronal networks abound, but the microneuronal bridge to cognition remains largely uncrossed. (Some progress in dealing with the cumulative states of neuronal networks of the amygdala does, however, suggest that progress is being made in this direction. See Nabavi et al., 2014)

Thus, for eminently practical combinatorial reasons, we are compelled to use macroneural, cumulative devices such as the functional Magnetic Resonance Imaging (fMRI), the Electroencephalographic (EEG), the Magnetoencephalographic (MEG), or other macroneural techniques for the foreseeable future. However, it must not be overlooked that, because these techniques pool or combine the neuronal responses into a global response measure, most of what is presumed by the Hebb theory to be critical necessary information about how the brain makes the mind is irretrievably lost.

The central question asked in this book is what kinds of theories are possible with information produced by these macroneural techniques? Is it possible to make some reasonable leaps of logic to overcome the degradation of the information inherent in this "lossy" data pooling? Is there enough residual information left that can help us to understand the magic by which material brain activity becomes intangible mental activity? To answer such questions, we must ask further questions of the nature of theory, of what empirical evidence is available, of what putative theories have already been forthcoming as well as of the technical complexities of the statistical methodology we now use. Our excursions along these pathways will, hopefully, lead us to a coherent and reasonable modern evaluation of the nature of theory in this important field of modern science as well as portend what the future may hold.

There are several general points that I should make at the outset of this discussion to avoid any confusion arising from the breadth of the mind-brain problem or my presentation.

1. The ultimate goal of this book is to examine what we know about the *macroneural* roots of cognition, where we are, and how far can we go towards an overarching theory using the associated methodology. Some of the barriers to explanation are general to science but some are specific to this level of cognitive neuroscience. (In a subsequent book, I plan to consider the microneuronal network approach.)

2. Cognition for me means high-level experiential processing. Sensory transmission codes and cognitive neural representation are different from those problems asked about cognition, and success in the former does not imply success in the latter.

3. My critique of brain imaging methods in cognitive studies does not deny the importance of devices such as the fMRI for anatomical and physiological studies and clinical use.

4. The argument that we do not and cannot have full and complete theories should not be interpreted as an argument that we should halt research in this field. There will be many wonderful and exciting discoveries in the future even though the mind-brain problem itself may not be cracked. There are

many useful contributions to be made even if a full and complete solution to the mind-brain problem turns out to be intractable.

5.   Many of the findings presented here either supporting or contraindicating macroneural theory building are not conclusive. Many are subject to interpretation, controversy, and methodological confusion about some of the most basic questions. However, the body of evidence that I find helpful is suggestive enough to challenge some widely held ideas.

6.   At the present time, my overall conclusion is that searching for the neural foundations of cognitive mechanisms (i.e., developing an overarching neuroreductionist theory of the mind using macroneural techniques) is a goal unlikely to be achieved. The use of fMRI systems to explain how the brain produces mental activity is simply being carried out at the wrong level of analysis. I agree with Page (2006), who asserted

> . . . the huge investment of time and money that has accompanied this trend [functional brain imaging] has not resulted in a corresponding theoretical advancement, at least with respect to cognitive psychological theory.
>
> *(p. 428)*

7.   The problem is currently exacerbated by the anticipated infusion of a billion or more dollars into research on what has been called the Brain Activity Map by Alivisatos et al. (2013) or the equally extravagantly funded Human Brain Project (Markram, 2006). Although it is certain that some new and valuable knowledge will come from such investments, the idea that that we can either map the brain or decode it at the microneuronal level is not supported by current research—in my opinion.

8.   I hope I am making a positive contribution by this analysis of the state of macrotheory in cognitive neuroscience. I feel strongly about the positions I have taken, but I also respect the quality of the work carried out by colleagues around the world, many of whom will not agree with some of the positions I have taken.

I could not finish this preface without making apologies to two groups of my fellow cognitive neuroscientists. The first includes those whose contributions I have either missed or simply glossed over. The sheer mass of publications in this field made it impossible for me to be aware of everything about which I should have known. I hope that the sample of topics I have chosen to highlight in this book is sufficient to support my main points.

The second group of cognitive neuroscientists to whom I must apologize includes those whose contributions I have interpreted differently than they originally did. This is a complex field in which even the most salient data may mean something different to different people.

ACKNOWLEDGMENTS

I officially retired a dozen years ago; nevertheless, during that time I have enjoyed the continued support of my two universities over this period. ASU's College of Engineering School of Computing, Informatics, Decision Systems Engineering, continues to provide me the necessities so that my work can proceed during the academic year. The Bekesy Laboratory of Neurobiology at the University of Hawaii has taken me in for the last 11 summers. I am deeply grateful to Patricia Couvillon, Lynn Hata, and my other colleagues and friends there for providing the same kind of intellectual environment in Honolulu as in Tempe.

Preparation of this book was partially supported by the US Army Research Institute for the Behavioral and Social Sciences under Contract Number W5J9CQ-12-C-0033. The views, opinions, and/or findings contained in this article are those of the author and shall not be construed as an official Department of the Army position, policy, or decision, unless so designated by other documents.

Most of all, I once again dedicate this book to the most important person in my life—my dear wife Mitchan, without whom nothing ever would have happened.

PROLOGUE

On the Antiquity of Cognitive Neuroscience

Cognitive neuroscience has often been presented as a brand new science that arose when the appropriate instrumentation became available. However, its antiquity is well established. Indeed, "published" reports of the relation between brain and mind are thousands of years old. Of course, the research tools (fingers) in those millennia were quite different and the significance inferred from the observations, as a result, also quite different. Whatever these differences, the earliest written records we have of mind-brain (actually of behavior-brain) relationships come from Egyptian medical papyri. One, in particular, the Edwin Smith Surgical Papyrus (Breasted, 1930) dated from the 17th century BCE, stands out because it is possibly the earliest written medical document of which copies still exist. However, its antiquity is only part of its interest to cognitive neuroscientists in the 21st century. It is important in the present context for another reason; it is probably the first writing that mentions an association between behavior and the brain—the first written expression of a primitive cognitive neuroscience. Consisting of a collection of case studies, the 20th case in the Smith papyrus describes how cranial damage could block speech and influence other motor functions—probably the first example of the science we now know as cognitive neuroscience.

Most of the cases described in this extraordinary document were aimed at establishing a medical prognosis associated with particular kinds of wound; in this case, a "wound to the temple"—a region of the skull that current-day insight permits us to presume overlays at least part of the speech and motor areas. It is in this regard that the significance of this antique document to mind-brain relationships was then and is still largely overlooked. Case 20, the one of special interest to us, is presented here verbatim according to the Breasted translation:

- Title: Instructions concerning a wound in his temple, penetrating to the bone, (and) perforating his temporal bone.

- Examination: If thou examinest a man having a wound in his temple, penetrating to the bone, (and) perforating his temporal bone, while his two eyes are blood shot, he discharges blood from both his nostrils, and a little drops; if thou puttest thy fingers on the mouth of that wound (and) he shudder exceedingly; if thou ask of him concerning his malady and he speak not to thee; while copious tears fall from both his eyes, so that he thrusts his hand often to his face that he may wipe both his eyes with the back of his hand as a child does, and knows not that he does so.
- Diagnosis: Thou shouldst say concerning him: "One having a wound in his temple, penetrating to the bone, (and) perforating his temporal bone; while he discharges blood from both his nostrils, he suffers with stiffness in his neck, (and) he is speechless. An ailment not to be treated."
- Treatment: Now when thou findest that man speechless, his [relief] shall be sitting; soften his head with grease, (and) pour [milk] into both his ears.

(Quoted from Breasted, 1930)

It is in these archaic words and sentences that the Egyptian physicians may have been the earliest to observe a specific relationship between the brain, mind, and behavior. The ancient Egyptian physicians who wrote this work reported that a stimulus—mechanical pressure—("puttest thy fingers on the mouth of that wound") led to both a behavioral effect ("he speak not to thee" or "shudder exceedingly") and a cognitive one ("knows not that he does so"). Should the Egyptian physicians have noted the close relationship between this particular head wound and speechlessness and convulsions, perhaps thinking about the role of the brain in the form of an anticipatory modern cognitive neuroscience might have had an earlier start than it did. Implicit in this Egyptian medical advice, of course is the persistent assumption by many cognitive neuroscientists that particular areas of the brain have specific functions.

Unfortunately, the significance of this early relation between brain and mind or behavior was not generalized to an appreciation that motor behavior and mental activity such as speech were regulated by the brain. To the Egyptians, despite this evidence, the heart remained the key organ embodying where the various entities of the mind resided.

This prologue to a discussion of mind-brain research and theory illustrates some important points. Most important is the powerful influence of methodology and situation on what kind of evidence and, thus, what kind of explanations would emerge. In the days of the Egyptian pharaohs, observations of the relationship between mental activity and brain activity depended on fortuitous injuries or trauma. Soldiers were regularly having their head damaged when swords and spears were the weapons of choice. The only "research" tools available to examine the exposed brain tissue were the physician's fingers. None of the esoteric paraphernalia used to manipulate or explore the resulting wounds in today's laboratories were available and so none of the currently popular explanatory ideas went unrecognized.

Throughout the history of the various sciences and perspectives about mind-brain relationships, the influence of available instrumentation (usually invented for use by some other science) remains definitive. This is a basic thesis of this book—that what and how we theorize about mind-brain relationships depends in large part on the measuring tools that are available at any time. Over the decades, one instrument or another has been of special import. Surgical intervention, electronic stimuli, microscopes, electronic high-gain amplifiers, electroencephalograms, and brain imagers have all come into play as they became available. Now powerful new computer techniques promise to open the door to a new generation of theories.

The absence of instruments that were able to study other aspects of what inspired speculation suggested might be the actual relationship between the brain and cognition severely inhibited understanding and theoretical progress. We did what we could with what we had. Thus, for the last three decades, during the heyday of functional magnetic resonance instruments, these devices dominated research protocols, the kind of evidence that could be gathered, and the macroscopic concepts and theories that could be derived.

However, for the last 30 years or so, there has been a general appreciation growing that the macroscopic signals from brain imaging equipment may not be seminal for overarching theories. Although brain images may correlate with cognitive functions, they are not conceptualized at the most germane level of analysis to inspire plausible explanations. In their place, a very different idea has grown—that the mind is encoded or represented or embodied in the networks of the vast number of microscopic neurons. As network thinking emerged and the tools for studying them proliferated, new theoretical postulates and theories emerged that had previously only been speculative.

I believe that cognitive neuroscience is at a point of transition—one in which our science is about to be transformed from one emphasizing the macroscopic level of analysis to one that will emphasize the microscopic scale. This is a fundamental change that will see brain imaging diminishing in importance to be replaced by multiple electrode arrays and extraordinary new computer systems. This book makes the case for this transition by presenting a critique of macroneural theories and prototheories. It will be followed, I hope, by a companion volume that examines the case against microneuronal theories.

1

WHAT IS A THEORY?

1.1 Toward a Definition of a Theory[1]

The crown jewels of any science are the integrative theories developed to consolidate a sometimes enormous and chaotic body of empirical evidence. As exciting are the fortuitous discoveries of new worlds, creatures, processes, or phenomena, each discovery becomes truly meaningful only in terms of the synoptic interpretations that are made of it and others like it. This is not meant to disparage exploration or well-controlled experimentation, but rather to emphasize that what we make collectively of such findings is the most important product of a science. Whether it is an understanding of the overall geography of a previously undiscovered land on Earth or in the cosmos or of the relations between animal species or between elemental materials, it is the syntheses of particular observations into general laws and principles and then the integration of these laws into overarching theory that characterize the great accomplishments of science.

Individual observations remain largely isolated and their meaning often cryptic, if not useless, without some kind of a conceptual framework. It is the cumulative and general impact of a body of knowledge, rather than the particulars of individual findings, that lead to prediction and control and all of the rest of the progress that comes from scientific inquiry. It is the ability to see general implications, as opposed to observed individual "facts," that provides the great payoff. It is this understanding and its application that eventually leads us to the betterment of life and the indescribable joy of discovering something universal about the world in which we live. Although individual experiments may excite, stimulate, and illuminate a dark corner of what had been ignorance, they mean nothing until their implications are made clear. Flames are charming and beautiful, but they took on a much deeper meaning when the general idea of combustion was explicated. When the spectrum of the light emitted from such a process permitted us to probe the nature of atomic structure, even deeper insights and theories became possible and science transcended from the mysterious to the comprehensible.

It is in this context that the word "theory" takes on such an especially important role in science. Nevertheless, it is probably among science's most misunderstood words. Debate concerning its meaning is ubiquitous among philosophers as well as among empirically oriented investigators. This is especially true in cognitive neuroscience—a science that has one foot in the tangible biochemistry and electrophysiology of nervous action and the other in the excruciatingly intangible phenomena of thought, consciousness, attention, perception, and emotion among other concepts of even less precise denotation.

In this book, I not only attempt to describe progress in current theory but also consider the constraints and barriers to theory building in cognitive neuroscience. After considerable research, I have some grave doubts about some of the theoretical goals in this field. My negative conclusion concerning the ultimate solubility of the mind-brain question is not unique or completely idiosyncratic. Others such as Rakover (2011) essentially came to the same conclusion. He cited a number of scholars (e.g., Dietrich & Hardcastle, 2005; Heil, 2003; Ludwig, 2003; McGinn, 1989; Palmer, 1999; Putnam, 1975) most of whom are philosophers, but all of whom express the same opinion—we have not yet explained how mental processes emerge from neural activity, and there is little hope that we will be able to do so in the immediate future! As a result, these scholars have come to be referred to as the "New Mysterians."

Cognitive neuroscientists, of course, have quite a different outlook about the ultimate solvability of the mind-brain problem, by which I mean specifically the search for a neuroreductionist explanation of how the brain produces the mind. Indeed, the entire corpus of their work is based on the presumption that not only is an explanation possible but also that we are making progress toward that goal. This is not to say that there is any ontological disagreement between current philosophers and cognitive neuroscientists about the physical basis of mind. Both groups mainly agree (no matter how much popular opinion may run against the idea) that the immaterial mind is nothing more or less than a function of the material brain. Both groups can accept the ontology of materialistic monism *in principle* while also accepting the epistemological *in practice* constraints on the task. To do otherwise is to flirt with a cryptic kind of dualism.

In such a context, if we are to talk sensibly about current developments in cognitive neuroscience, it is essential that we are as precise as possible about what we mean by the word "theory." In an earlier work (Uttal, 2005), I attempted to define the term by an exhaustive search of the literature. It did not take long to discover that there was a great diversity of meanings that had been attached to the word over the centuries. Some are pejorative (one common use of the word "theory" is as a substitute for knowledge), as a designation of our ignorance rather than of our understanding. In this context, "theory" is used to imply unsupported speculation as in, "Oh, that is only a theory."

Similarly, the word "theory" is also sometimes used as a prevailing, informal statement of some presumed, but unsupported, relationship. For example, "the theory is that most children have a natural affinity for music." Whether this statement is true, the scientific literature justifying such a "theory" is controversial, to say the least. This "theoretical" assertion, like many other such conjectures about human nature, is far less strongly substantiated than we would wish. The meaning of the word "theory" in this case is more akin to a preliminary assumption, hypothesis, or premise than a general law.

In other contexts, theory is used as the beginning, and not the end, of a scientific inquiry. Here it is frequently mistakenly confused with "hypothesis." Not all hypotheses, of course, are theory free; they may well have developed from a previous synthesis—a previous prototheory or hypothesis that offered a preliminary understanding of a collection of observations.

Hypotheses are, at best, limited intermediate steps by means of which prototheories and theories can be invoked and tested.

A prototheory is defined as an intermediate step between observational data and a true, complete, explanatory theory. Prototheories include organized collections of data as well as preliminary interpretations, simulations, and correlational statements. Although usually "explaining" very little, they have the possibility of stimulating subsequent steps towards overarching explanatory theories.

Thus, a hypothesis still does not represent the ideal goal of a unifying synthesis. Of course, theoretical constructs can be tested by playing the role of "hypotheses" in experiments; however, the prototypical experiment in such a case is usually framed in something more akin to a limited question than as an overarching theory. For example, the measurement of the deflection of light by the gravitational attraction of the sun by Dyson, Eddington, and Davidson (1920) was a test of a hypothesis (light would be bent by gravity) that then could be applied as a test of a theory (Einstein's general relativity theory). By itself, the observation was of minor practical significance (no human endeavor was obviously changed by the observation itself). In the context of the theory of which it was a test, confirmation of the predictive hypothesis was world changing.

I sought an answer to the nature of a theory in my earlier book by quoting from the *Merriam-Webster Collegiate Dictionary* (2000). What I found was a number of definitions, some of which came close to my use whereas others were really nothing more than colloquialisms. [The bracketed responses are my own.]

1. the analysis of a set of facts in their relation to one another. [GOOD!]
2. abstract thought: SPECULATION [TERRIBLE!]
3. the general or abstract principles of a body of fact, a science, or an art <music *theory*> [GOOD!]
4a. a belief, policy, or procedure proposed or followed as the basis of action <her method is based on the *theory* that all children want to learn> (b): an ideal or hypothetical set of facts, principles, or circumstances—often used in the phrase *in theory* <in *theory*, we have always advocated freedom for all> [TRIVIAL!]
5. a plausible or scientifically acceptable general principle or body of principles offered to explain phenomena <wave *theory* of light> [GOOD!]
6a. a hypothesis assumed for the sake of argument or investigation [POOR!] (b): an unproved assumption: CONJECTURE [POOR!] (c): a body of theorems presenting a concise systematic view of a subject <*theory* of equations> [GOOD!]

Synonyms see HYPOTHESIS² [POOR AND MISLEADING!]

My purpose in pointing out the variety of usages of the word "theory" is to lay the foundation for the meaning of the word as I use it throughout the rest of this book. The most important point to be made explicit at this point in our discussion is that *an assemblage of data does not a theory make*. That is, no matter how extensive may be a body of empirical knowledge, it is just a collection of observations until organized into a coherent story. By "coherent" I mean that the individual observations must collectively imply some general synthesis. Only when the similarities and relationships are highlighted and the general principles extracted does the beginning of a theory emerge.

A theory is an integrated interpretation of a body of related empirical evidence. As such, a theory incorporates or summarizes a body of observations by extracting general principles, rules, and laws implied by the data. Theories come in many types—some mathematically formal and some ambiguously verbal—but all of which transcend the particular to illuminate the general. In this book, I emphasize the neuroreductionist approach, in particular, at the macroneural level.

There are a variety of theories about the how the brain makes the mind, but none is unique or dominant. Some theories are purely descriptive, using logical and mathematical frameworks to depict the behavior of a system. Some dote on predictability as their central idea. Some are patently reductive, invoking and synthesizing data that hopefully bridge the huge conceptual and empirical gap between the neural and the mental.

Philosophers (e.g., Hesse, 1967) invoke a hierarchy of observations, laws, and theories. The first being the raw data, the second being generalities inferred from the data, and the third incorporating the laws into a system that may have reductive, deductive, or predictive implications. Throughout this hierarchy, there is a consolidation and simplification of the world as we observe it into ever more general ideas. Thus a law, however general, is not a theory until it is combined with other laws. Throughout this process, there is the progressive consolidation from particulars to ever more encompassing generalities.

For example, Guthrie (1946) asserted the following:

> A flood of new publications is not automatically a flood of new facts. In addition, it may include many facts that do not contribute materially to the science of psychology. Collections of facts are not science. They are the material out of which science can grow, but they are only the raw material of science, and sometimes they are not even that.
>
> *(p. 3)*

The essence of my use of the word "theory" is that a theory is a collection of general laws and principles that transcend and enlarge on the meaning of the empirical observations on which the theory was based. The particular emphasis that I make as a cognitive neuroscientist is that the cognitive should in principle be explained (or an effort made towards explanation) by linking the languages of psychology and neurophysiology.

A common theme expressed by those of us who have seriously considered the issue—what is a theory?—is that the primary attribute of a theory is that it is comprehensive, inclusive, and integrative of the findings of many experiments. The metaphorical image to which a theory is often compared is of a pyramid, in which the lower levels represent the particular data, findings, or observations, and the upper levels are increasingly more inclusive of a variety of general rules, laws, and principles—in other words, the most general apex of the pyramid represents the theory.

To the extent that we can predict the future, it will most likely be discovered that that the level of brain activity that will ultimately emerge as the foundation of cognition is that of neuronal network interactions at the microneuronal level (Hebb, 1949). Macroneural signals such as those obtained with an fMRI system may pool, sum, and combine these salient neuronal (cellular) interactions and thus obliterate the information that is necessary for theory development.

By *macroneural,* I refer to neural processes and responses that are the summed, pooled, or cumulative effects of a large number of neurons distributed over extended regions of the brain. By *microneuronal,* I refer to the neural processes of single neurons or to networks of neurons in which the identity and function of the individual neurons are preserved.

There are two main barriers to the development of neuroreductionist theories. The first, inhibiting macroneural theory, is that any inconsistency between cognitive and neural activities may reflect the fact that macroneural electrophysiological signals are actually unrelated to cognitive processes, but are, instead, statistical artifacts based on inadequate sample size or too liberal p-values. The possibility that we are reading order into what is actually a stochastic process is not too far-fetched, given the recent contributions of Thyreau et al. (2012) and Gonzalez-Castillo et al. (2012) that are discussed extensively in Chapter 5. If their arguments and findings turn out to be valid when replicated, it would be a major problem for any theory depending on some form of localization, for then there would be no robust evidence of separable, localizable brain regions in particular places—a major postulate of current cognitive neuroscience. Data sets from brain imaging experiments would have to be considered as cumulative expressions of a myriad of components in a complex system rather than as prototheories. Under some conditions, particularly those of brain-like systems, this may pose intractable barriers to theory building.

The second major barrier affects putative microneuronal theories. It may be that the number of neurons and the complexity of the neuronal networks are such that the combinatorial problem they specify to understand their cognitive functions may pose, for the foreseeable future, intractable computational or data-handling obstacles.

It is uncertain how profound are these barriers. If consistency is to be found when comparable experiments are replicated, then at least the raw materials of a prototheory may be present.[3] The term "prototheory" refers specifically to a body of data, or a loose interpretation of them, that does not meet the criteria of generality and synoptic convergence required of a true or complete explanatory theory. Instead, prototheories are often little more than simple restatements, tabulations, collections, or organizations of the empirical data.

It is not entirely clear what constitutes a prototheory. Nor, for that matter, is it necessarily true that just a body of accumulated data, no matter how voluminous, would ipso facto constitute a theory. The ideal theory, as I have already noted, goes beyond the data to tease out the generalities and universals in a manner that transcends the corpus of empirical evidence.

Obviously, the converse is also true—just as a scientific theory must be based on relevant empirical evidence, a putative summary based on flimsy or nonexistent evidence does not deserve the appellation of theory. It may be a speculation, belief, metaphorical model, or conjecture, but not a "theory" in the more restricted sense used here.

Despite these caveats, modern neurosciences, crossing levels of analyses and invoking what might be considered to be various kinds of primitive prototheories, are common these days. Such "theories" often misunderstand the nature of the gap between an ontological postulate that the mind is a function of the brain, on the one hand, and the epistemological constraints on what we can understand about this complex organ, on the other.

Within this general context, it is clear that there are many criteria with which theories and prototheories can be classified. A mini-taxonomy of theoretical prototypes and theories, only some of which rise to the level of theory, is now presented. Admittedly, the proposed dichotomy between prototheories and theories is arbitrary but is useful as a means of making the point that not all "theories" are actually reductive or explanatory theories.

Prototheories

- Biomarkers
- Typologies
- Taxonomies
- Correlations (With and without predictive powers)
- Recapitulations of Data
- Metaphors
- Cladistics
- Translations of the Data to a Different Language (e.g., from a psychophysical observation to neural terminology)
- Data Extraction, Manipulation, and Analysis Methods Imitating Theories

Theories

- Descriptive Theories
  - Formal Theories
  - Control Systems
  - Mechanical Models
- Reductive Theories
  - Explanatory Theories

Although this framework is obviously incomplete and many other categories and criteria of what is a "theory" or a "prototheory" could be invoked to classify them, this table, at least, provides a usable schema for the present discussion. They all make an implicit assertion that may be at the least a precursor (i.e., a prototheory) of future understanding. To identify the limited scope of "theory" I intend to consider in this book, I provide the following nutshell definition.

A neuroreductive theory of cognition is based on the postulate that it may ultimately be possible to show how the tangible neural components and functions of the brain produce the intangible functions of the mind. Like all theories, it must transcend particular results to produce general syntheses. Preferably, it must "explain" rather than merely "describe" or even "predict." Whether a true and complete neuroreductionist theory of cognition is a realistic goal is yet to be determined.

1.2 Prototheories

Some cognitive neuroscientific prototheories eschew any direct or causal relation between the neurophysiological state and cognition. Instead, their role is simply to serve as an indicator that may be useful in meeting some clinical need. For example, physiological "biomarkers" may signify a relationship between a neurophysiological measurement and a clinical abnormality, but make no claim to any direct causal or explanatory relationship between the physiological indicator and a disease state. As such, they fulfill the same role as does a thermometer: As a general, but indirect, indicator of underlying organic dysfunction whose real origins may not be directly determinable.

Biomarkers may be very simple (e.g., the temperature) or very complicated (e.g., the polygraphic response of which is supposedly capable of detecting deception, Larson, 1921). The combined sphygmomanometer, plethysmograph, and electrodermal responses have been frequently and unjustifiably used as biomarkers for deception despite the fact that there is no well-established linkage between telling a lie and any of the physiological measures recorded by these devices (Adler, 2007).

In some more sophisticated cases, some preliminary relationships among the "specimens" of a collection may be established. Prototheories of this kind might be called taxonomies or typologies—an initial step in the organization of the data that may ultimately lead to full-blown theories. They deserve to be called prototheories because they often provide a heuristic or highlight some aspect or relationship of a finding that may lead to a more formal kind of theory.

Another stage in the development of a prototheory is one in which numerical correlations are established between cognitive processes and neurophysiological states. Such a process adds information and may also lead the way to a theory; however, such numerical correlations are not tantamount to causal explanations (Yule, 1926). Correlations between stimuli and responses, by themselves, are not definitive in terms of the internal functional relationships except in an indirect way; they merely describe the interconnected nature of the system.

A number of cognitive neuroscientists including Koch and Greenfield (2007) have suggested that the goal of current cognitive neuroscience is solely to determine the Neural Correlates of Consciousness. Whether a system based on correlations between vaguely defined consciousness and inconsistent brain responses can possibly lead to explanations of particular mind-brain relationships remains problematic. Unfortunately, it may be that this is the best we can do—to develop a correlative or descriptive cognitive neuroscience rather than an explanatory one—but the hope is that some progress may be made towards a full and complete theoretical explanation of mental processes. There may be some more complete descriptive, explanatory, or reductive theory lurking in the future, but there is little evidence of progress being made on the basis of correlations alone—the bridges between correlation and causation being so fragile. In short, if Koch and Greenfield are correct, cognitive neuroscience is mainly a nonreductive empirical, as opposed to a theoretical, science.

Cognitive neuroscience prototheories come in many forms; some of them are nothing more or less than complex *aide memoires* without explanatory value but useful in metaphorically conceptualizing a problem area. Of course, in the real cognitive neuroscience experimental world, experiments are usually guided by some kind of hypotheses based on a variety of insights. However, these hypotheses usually turn out to be tests of very specific questions (e.g., hypotheses) rather than tests of theories.

The point is that by designating something as a theory does not automatically make it such. Many so called "neurotheories" have proliferated as the seductive[4] nature of brain images has made its way from our scientific culture to that of the mundane world. In recent years, a host of new "neurosciences" have been proposed, based on purported links between both macroneural and microneuronal neurophysiological data, on the one hand, and various aspects of human cognition or social interaction, on the other. Many of these new "sciences," (e.g., Neuroeconomics) however, are based on an extrapolation from a very limited database or, all too often, on none at all.

In general, the most effective criticism of these novel pseudosciences is that they do not reflect the great gap between the ontological postulate that the brain is "the organ of the mind" and the epistemological fact that we have not built nor are likely to build the kind of intellectual bridges that could possibly cross the gap between possibility and actuality.

A number of scholars have argued generally against the trend of attaching the prefix "Neuro" to almost any other field of intellectual endeavor. To do so suggests that theoretical progress has been made when, in fact, none exists. This has led to a wildly hyperbolic effort to capitalize commercially on what is still largely unknown. For example, in an editorial in the *Journal of Cognitive Neuroscience,* Farah (2008) identifies commercial organizations *Amen Clinic, FKF Applied Research, Cephos,* and *No Lie MRI* as being among the many commercial exploiters of extravagant and scientifically unsupportable claims in nouveaux fields such as Neuropolitics and Neurolaw, or even as new approaches to psychotherapy. Further arguments against the casual creation of novel neurosciences based on inadequate basic science have been made by Legrenzi and Umiltà (2011). They pejoratively express these new developments as alternate forms of "Neuromania." Tallis (2011) also attacked the idea that brain images are informative indicators of complex cognitive processes. Furthermore, Wastell and White (2012) also argued that current child-rearing practice is overly influenced by questionable neuroscientific findings.

With this introduction in hand, we can now turn to some specific examples of prototheories.

Biomarkers

A modern form of questionable biomarker can be found in the work of Redcay and Courchesne (2005), who argued that the size of the brain was an indicator of autism. Although the exact neural cause of autism remains unclear, it seems unlikely that raw brain size could be anything more than a biomarker—it has no explanatory value in understanding the causes of the dysfunction. More seriously, the data supporting this hypothetical relation are inconsistent. (For an authoritative summary of the discrepancies in this field, see Brambilla et al., 2003.)

The historical search for a biomarker for an illness such as schizophrenia has occupied researchers for many decades without success. Recently, Javitt, Spencer, Thaker, Winterer, and Hajos (2008) reviewed the potential use of a number of proposed neurophysiological "biomarkers" including the EEG, P-300 ERP, and fMRI without finding any one that could presently be used as a diagnostically useful indicator of this disabling mental condition. Although they were enthusiastic supporters of the hope that a neural biomarker for schizophrenia would eventually be found someday, they acknowledged that the search for such a physiological biomarker has so far been fruitless. Perhaps the current state of the ultimate quest on which Javitt and his colleagues had embarked could be best summed up by their words "[the] underlying genetic and neuronal abnormalities [of schizophrenia] are largely unknown" (p. 68).

Indeed, it may be that this quest may be another ill-defined one. Like so many other cognitive dysfunctions, beyond the ultimate generalization of mind-brain equivalence, the word "schizophrenia" may not be a biologically coherent category that exists only in the vagaries of psychiatric nosology. Unfortunately, in such a context, a comprehensive theoretical explanation of this debilitating disease is not even on the horizon.

Despite the fact that no robust neural biomarker is yet known for any of the other equally poorly defined mental dysfunctions that currently seem to be almost epidemic (e.g., autism, hyperactivity syndromes, posttraumatic disorders, and a disordered list of mental illnesses and confused social relationships[5]), this atheoretical approach dominates current psychotherapeutic research efforts because of the failure of the search for deep understanding of the actual causal factors. Furthermore, there may be other reasons for this inability to find any neural activity correlated with these complex mental dysfunctions. They are all examples of spectrum disorders that probably involve different combinations of causes, symptoms, and dysfunctions. Nevertheless, as a result of this limit on both definitional and diagnostic precision, it seems unlikely that the search for this kind of biomarker is likely to succeed. Nevertheless, as shown by Singh and Rose (2009), there has been an almost exponential rise in publications in which the word "biomarker" is used in recent years as new neurophysiological measures have become available.

The concept of the biomarker, as described here, is a prototheoretical approach to providing indicators of neural and psychological disorders. However, if further investigated, biomarkers can become a precursor of a real integrative theory. Should an acceptably high correlation be established between one of these dysfunctional states and a neurophysiological measure, this could serve as a heuristic or guide that could possibly lead to a more comprehensive theory of abnormal mind-brain relationships. Unfortunately, at the present time, few of the currently proposed biomarkers relating brain activity and cognitive pathologies seem to be able to gain traction in the way that would make us want to designate them even as a prototheory in the sense used in this book.

Typologies

A typology is defined as a simple classification system in which the specimens are organized according to certain identifiable similarities in structure, behavior, color, or other properties; in other words, a system based on similarities of properties. The traditional collections of butterflies, minerals, flowers (or, as some would argue, cognitive processes, experiences, and feelings as defined by psychologists) might represent typologies depending on how they were arranged. The pattern of observed relations in the properties of the items in the collection itself may be its own raison d'être. Although no formal rules may guide constructions of the types, the similarities among the specimens may subsequently stimulate the development of an ordered theoretical perspective as was so clearly evidenced by the collections of such theoretical scientists as Charles Darwin (1809–1882) and Alfred R. Wallace (1823–1913). It was the implicit order (e.g., slight variations that were due to geographical distributions) of the properties of their respective collections that led each of them to develop the grandest biological theory of all—organic evolution. However, before the formulations of their respective theories, for which they now appropriately share independent authorship, came the typological collections made by each of them in their roles as field naturalists. It is remarkable how similar are their scientific biographies as well as their earth-shaking conclusions.

Psychology is replete with such typologies that have not yet contributed to the formulation of an integrated theoretical system. Indeed, it is not too much of a stretch to argue that the subject matter of psychology is best described as a typology into which observations are categorized into such "types" as emotion, learning, and attention based on differences in experimental protocols. Among the best known psychological typologies are the hundreds of types of learning that have been identified by psychologists since the time of Hermann Ebbinghaus (1850–1909).

Taxonomies

To point out a classic example of a pregnant prototheoretical typology, when Dmitri Mendeleev (1834–1907) arranged the table of chemical elements in a way that highlighted the similarities and differences among the elements, the stage was set for the development of modern atomic physics based as it is on the functional properties of the different materials. Subsequent evidence led to the discovery of basic particles such as the electron in 1897 by J. J. Thomson (1856–1940), the proton in 1917 by Ernest Rutherford (1871–1937), and the neutron in 1932 by James Chadwick (1891–1974). These empirical discoveries were rounded out by Niels Bohr (1885–1962) who proposed a full-blown theory of the atom consisting of a central positively charged nucleus populated by protons and neutrons and surrounded by negatively charged orbital electrons. This ultimate theory made the different properties of the elements meaningful.

Observational taxonomies of the chemistry of the atomic elements thus provided the impetus for the development of a continuing series of ever more complex theories of the atom. The process fed back on itself as the atomic structural ideas provided what is still the most powerful and comprehensive explanation of the chemical behavior of the elements based on atomic-level attractions and repulsions. Subsequently, the entire science of physics was nearly (but not quite yet) unified in the concepts of the "standard model." Psychology, unfortunately, has not yet provided a unifying taxonomy, much less a theory of behaviors except in the most narrowly defined domains.[6]

Correlations

Another means by which typological collections can move beyond taxonomies is by establishing a quantitative measure of the relationships between the properties of the collected items. This is the correlative method implemented within the context of statistical analyses. The idea of numerical estimates of relationships—correlations—was first developed by Francis Galton (1822–1911) and further developed by Karl Pearson (1857–1936) and G. Udny Yule (1871–1951) and remains especially relevant in current cognitive neuroscience. Both Pearson and Yule were very concerned about the potential misunderstanding that *correlations* were tantamount to *explanations* of the causal influences underlying some phenomenon; in other words, that correlation might be mistakenly interpreted to imply causation and that those tables of correlations might be accepted as explanatory theories.

Aldrich (1995) also noted that the classic misunderstanding that "correlated variables . . . [depended] on common causes" (p. 364) identified by Pearson and Yule is still common in psychology. In historical fact, it is also likely that such an assumption is still rampant throughout cognitive neuroscience as well as psychology. It was to Yule (1911) that the following quotation is attributed:

> Any interpretation of the meaning of an [correlative] association is necessarily hypothetical, and the number of possible alternative hypotheses is in general considerable.
>
> *(p. 42)*

This statement parallels a stronger assertion by Moore (1956), an automata theorist, who argued:

> Theorem 2: Given any machine S and any multiple experiments performed on S, there exist other machines experimentally indistinguishable from S for which the original experiment would have had the same outcomes.
>
> *(p. 140)*

On a closely related issue, Aldrich (1995) also reported that both Pearson and Yule had developed concerns that "spurious" or "illusory" correlations could be created all too easily if two time series, for example, were both monotonic in the same direction. Both real and illusory correlations of this kind could lead investigators to infer functional relationships where none actually existed.

Both arguments—correlation should not be interpreted as causation and illusory correlations are all too likely—set the stage for a stronger and more general assertion; namely that all mathematical models, including stochastic and behavioral ones, are neutral with regard to underlying mechanisms. This is not a trivial point. It is a major barrier to reductive theory development throughout cognitive neuroscience. It asserts that, in principle, it is impossible to validate any mathematical model beyond its descriptive role because any particular mathematical model can be implemented in what may be an infinite number of ways.

Neutrality is a synonym for *underdetermined*. Both words allude to the fact that neither behavior nor mathematics contains enough information to distinguish among a multitude of possible underlying mechanisms or processes.

The main reason for the neutrality of mathematical or behavioral descriptions is the one highlighted by both Yule and Moore: There are a huge number of alternative internal mechanisms that could produce the same behavior or derive the same theorem. Systems of correlations, therefore, are not fully functioning theories any more than are taxonomies; they simply represent quantitative estimates of the degree of the relations between items in the collection, hopefully in a way that might suggest similarities and reductive explanations among the specimens and, thus, could lead to theories in the exemplary manner achieved with the Bohr atom.

Obviously, misinterpretations, strategic errors, or simple calculation errors in statistical analysis can also have major effects on cognitive neuroscience theories. The implications for theory are deeply troubling when so much of modern cognitive neuroscience is based on highly variable responses that can be identified only by elaborate statistical methods that were developed in an effort to overcome poor signal-to-noise relations. Throughout cognitive and neuroscientific studies, thresholds for significance are relatively low in any case—.05 being an arbitrary and loose value frequently used.[7] Should we also have to account for 18% calculation errors, 15% significance errors, or 50% strategic errors cited by Bakker and Wicherts (2011), serious questions arise about how well these cognitive neuroscience prototheories will be able to evolve into valid and comprehensive theories. However, the calculation errors may be less serious than the conceptual errors in assuming that any mathematical model can be successfully used as a reductive theory of cognitive processes, a point made very effectively by Miller (2010). In short, no matter how successfully a predictive mathematical model may be, it cannot uniquely define internal structure.

Recapitulations of Data

Another form of prototheory especially common in cognitive neuroscience is actually a cryptic recapitulation or restatement of the findings in a slightly different language than that in which they were originally measured. For example, most current fMRI experiments conclude their presentation with some kind of a statement of the locations or spatial distribution of activation areas elicited by the assigned cognitive stimuli or tasks. Sentences such as "Area A" (or, more likely these days, "Areas A, B . . . AND Z") "were shown to be significantly activated during certain cognitive processes" typically represent the final prototheoretical conclusion of many experimental reports these days. Thus, data becomes theory as in, areas A, B, . . . AND Z *are* the brain locations mediating that cognitive process.

In recent years, there has been a concerted effort to go beyond this simplistic theoretical association of place and function to more elaborate analysis of brain areas and how they may interact (see as pertinent examples the works by Friston et al,

2007; Poldrack, Mumford, & Nichols, 2011; and Sporns, 2011). Their empirical observations (which areas are activated) become the neural equivalents of the particular cognitive processes. Many other experiments that claim to be offering a theory are, in fact, only testing a hypothesis or are just recapitulating the observed data. Important logical links are missing in such a sequence, however—most notably answers to the basic question, how does an ensemble of activation areas encode cognition?

Metaphors

Another way to transform the data obtained in an experiment into a seemingly theoretical statement is by means of a metaphor. By a metaphor, I am referring to a description summarizing opinions of how a system is organized using the words and symbols from some other domain of discourse. The words of a metaphor might, thus, be drawn from a completely different context than the one under investigation. For example, Broadbent (1958) used the metaphor of a mechanical funnel to clarify the limited nature of our attention span. In this case, the metaphorical nature of this kind of model was clear—the two kinds of entity simply seemed to behave in an analogous manner.

In other instances, however, the metaphorical language might even come from the same domain as that being represented, and the fact that a prototheory is but a metaphor may not be evident. Thus, for example, a representation of the brain as an aggregation of localized, function-specific nodes may actually be a simplifying metaphor for whatever is the current view of brain organization. Such a description may appear superficially to be a reductive theory of the brain activity, but, in actuality, it may be nothing more than a metaphor or, even worse, just a cryptic recapitulation of the empirical findings as just discussed. In this instance, neural language is used to "vividly express" certain properties of a neural system when, in fact, the physical nature of the metaphor bears only a distant relation to the actual organization and properties of the system under study. Thus, a metaphor may be nothing more than a statement of the prevailing opinion or consensus of how the mind-brain system might be organized.

For example, at the outset of brain imaging research in cognitive neuroscience in the 1990s, the prevailing metaphor was the phrenological one. All of the experimental strategies and paradigms were based on the idea that psychological faculties or functions could be divided into modules and processes that were executed by comparable function-specific, narrowly localized brain regions. As new data accumulated, the prevailing metaphor changed to one of functional interactions between hypothetical cognitive modules at the psychological level and multiple distributed non-function-specific regions of the brain. Thus, although the prevailing metaphor changed, it did no more than restate the contemporary findings in the language of the currently dominant perspective. We were, at that time, still at a level of "barefoot empiricism" in which the data were just reported, albeit with little synthesis. It is arguable whether any such viewpoint, perspective, metaphor, or whatever one wishes to call it, even deserved the approbation prototheory.

Cladistics

There is another level of prototheory that deserves brief notice at this point. Not all of the prototheories I have discussed so far are simple tabulations or recapitulations of the data. The correlative method is a quantitative approach that seeks to define the relations among items in a collection. One of the most formidable of the new correlation methods is cladistics, a methodology that uses common features of a collection of observations to produce a relational taxonomy of the heritage of a group of specimens.

Modern cladistics was originally conceived of by Hennig (1966) under the name "Phylogenetic Systematics," a term later replaced by the term cladistics. The word now has come to be associated specifically with Hennig's computational method of organizing a collection of entities into their relationships such that a common ancestor can be identified. The main goal of the cladistics approach is to remove subjectivity from the development of genealogies of this kind. To do so, however, required substantial computer power—this being the main reason that its development was so recent. The output of the computation would be a "clade"—a grouping consisting of a common ancestor and all of its descendents.

Cladistical computations are closely related to evolutionary theory because they both depend on common hereditary characteristics of the items in the collection. However, they do not represent anything beyond a prototheory of evolution; it would require an astute observer to make the intellectual leap from even the most precisely defined clade to a reductive explanation of the mechanisms of how the clades emerged.

The main criterion for organizing the clade is one of parsimony; that is, the simplest tree of relationships that can fit the data is assumed to be the best taxonomy. Ideally, the output of such a computation offered by a formal method such as cladistics is a precise, quantitatively based statement of the relations between items in the clade in a more objective and efficient way than that produced by an insightful human taxonomist or by simple correlations. It is another example of a prototheory, a systematic method of organizing the data that may provide a heuristic for the development of a theory in the future; but, at best, it is not a reductive explanation of mechanisms and processes, just a description of relationships. Although complex and objective, cladistics is mainly a formal means of organizing the data and, like so many other prototheories, can only lead indirectly to explanations of process.

1.3 Simulation

Simulation is another approach that can be included in the rubric of "proto-theory." In this context, we must make a distinction between mimicry and explanation. By so doing, we appreciate that a simulation is constructed to reproduce or mimic some kind of behavior (mathematically, by computer programs, or even by mechanical models). However, it may do so by mechanisms and processes that have little or nothing to do with the actual underlying neurophysiological mechanisms producing that behavior in an organism. A second order differential equation, for example, may model the frequency of an oscillatory pendulum, totally ignoring the material nature of the forces producing the behavior. Indeed, a charging capacitor, the dynamics of predator-prey populations, or the movement of the pendulum may be modeled by exactly the same mathematical equation despite the fact that they are based on completely different physical mechanisms. No matter how closely the simulated behavior may match the real behavior, the results are entirely neutral. Often, the properties and capabilities of the devices (e.g., computers) used to mimic the behavior are the determining factors rather than the neural properties of the brain itself.

A distinction can be drawn, therefore, between simulations and explanatory theories. Both may share a common mathematical structure; however, their respective goals may be quite different. A simulation is typically aimed at developing a system that behaves in the same manner as the system under investigation. To do so, it may invent, infer, or speculate about the internal components of the systems necessary to provide the desired behavior. It may also draw upon processes that are known to be useful from other fields. For example, algorithms or devices (e.g., a shift register) can be applied from computer science that have no known equivalent biological function in order to produce a desired behavior.

Unfortunately, because the simulated behavior is underdetermined, and there are many possible mechanisms that are mathematical duals or can mimic each other's behavior, simply constructing a simulation, even a functionally successful one, may be remote from a true explanation of how the behavior originates. Examples of simulations produced by computational neuroscientists that are designed to mimic cognitive behavior but are not specifically explanations of the emergence of mental activity have been reviewed and discussed by de Garis, Chen, Goertzel, and Lian (2010). These reviewers make several important contributions. Among the most salient is the realization that many of these simulations may not be neurobiologically relevant. That is, a simulation, even one involving over 100,000 neuromimes (computer algorithms simulating the behavior of neurons) might have a limited or nonexistent contribution to make to the mind-brain problem. A more common benefit is a contribution to computer technology; for example, the creation of an algorithm or processor that enhances the speed of executing some otherwise ponderous, time-consuming program. A notable example in this context is the invention of the Fast Fourier Transform (Cooley & Tukey, 1965).

A general suggestion emerging as one reads the de Garis et al. (2010) review of what is now called "computational neuroscience" is the cavalier manner in which the language of cognitive neuroscience has been appropriated for the purposes of "brain-like" simulations. Programs of this type do not typically simulate the highly irregular manner in which brain components are interconnected. To the contrary, by necessity, their modules are interconnected by a few types (or even one type) of "tracts." This is quite unlike the irregular and idiosyncratic manner in which the components of real brains are interconnected. Yet the phrase "brain-like computers" is ubiquitous throughout all of these discussions regardless of whether their computer models share anything beyond the basic postulate that brains and computers are both networks of many components. The key property of a brain that makes it so adaptive and responsive probably has more to do with the heterogeneity of the interconnections, and these may not be adequately simulated for what are eminently practical reasons—there are far too many of them.

A follow-up article (Goertzel, Lian, Arel, de Garis, & Chen, 2010) introduced a striking discrepancy between two meanings of the phrase "artificial brain." In the original article (de Garis, Chen, Goertzel, & Lian, 2010), an artificial brain was a vast network of neuronal-like elements interconnected in a relatively regular order—the more synthetic neurons that could be manipulated, the better. In the follow-up article, Goertzel et al.'s attention shifted to a completely different level of analysis—"cognitive architectures." Words such as "neurons" and concepts such as neuroreductionism have disappeared almost entirely and have been replaced by hypothetical constructs such as the "retrieval buffer," a concept introduced from computer technology; in other words, by symbolic structures that had no neural referents, only behavioral, psychological, and functional entities. Models of this type are not so much "inspired by the brain" as inspired by behavior. The language of the discussion had, thus, shifted from that of microneuronal interactions of de Garis et al. to mimicry at the behavioral, cognitive, or psychological level. Goertzel's colleagues are no longer carrying out an exercise in neuroreductionism but exploring a kind of theory that has little or no relevance to the neural domain—the range of topics included in this book. Their review is of theories that are psychologically or behaviorally inspired, not neurally. The central point to be made here from this transition, however, is that even a perfectly fitting simulation precisely reproducing the behavior of some system may do so by mechanisms and processes that have little to do with the actual neurobiological causes of that behavior.

Because simulations and theories overlap to a certain degree (both may represent the behavior of a complex system), it is often difficult to precisely distinguish between these two categories beyond their intent. Simulations can be carried out at many different levels of analysis; one is reminded of the large-scale studies of the neuronal network types just discussed. The primary goal of a simulation is to understand how large arrays of components interact. Although occasionally clothed in the language of neurophysiology ("we are going to build a brain") it is more likely that investigators in this field are actually concerned with the computational properties of very large and uniformly interconnected networks that may be very different from those of the brain. Simulations of this kind, once past the linguistic obeisance of denoting them as neural or brain models, eventually can claim only that they have ferreted out the properties of large-scale networks; but it is a stretch to assert that they have built a "brain." The same research could as well have been carried out and the same results obtained without intent that they were simulations of real biological functions.

1.4 Theories

So far I have suggested that it is not appropriate to designate any of the previously discussed prototheories as even approximations to complete explanatory theories. The mind-brain problem, it is generally accepted, remains refractory at least and impossible to solve at worst. This brings us to the next step in this discussion: If the prototheories just discussed are not theories, what is a theory? If we cannot yet provide such a theory, can we at least see some of the properties of what a neuroreductionist theory of mental activity might be? In an earlier part of this chapter, I made a step towards a definition of such a theory in terms of its ability to generalize the results of many salient observations into a comprehensive, unifying, synoptic statement. That is, it must not be simply a statement (or a cryptic restatement) of the data—as most current cognitive neuroscience prototheories appear to be—but something that transcends individual experiments. Thus, a theory is characterized to me most of all by its ability to encompass a wide variety of empirical observations into a unified statement of general rules and principles. In other words, it must be the tip of the pyramid of relevant scientific description and interpretation.[8] When the data being synthesized relate neural data and cognitive process, then it would be fair to distinguish it as a neuroreductionist theory. When the data are forthcoming from the domain of large regions of the brain, then it is appropriate to distinguish it as a macroneural theory.

   I have chosen to use a dichotomous classification system to characterize what I believe are the various theoretical types currently being proposed in cognitive neurosciences. Theories of the mind-brain relation (along with those of any other science) seem to me to fall into two categories—descriptive and reductive. I appreciate that these two words are used in a multitude of ways by my colleagues, so it is important that I make my use clear at the outset of this discussion.[9]

Descriptive Theories

By a descriptive theory, I refer to one in which the behavior of the system under investigation is represented in words, rules, or equations without any effort to reduce the functions of that system to lower (in our case, neural) levels of analysis or the components thereof. Indeed, the key idea in this mode of theory building is that description is intrinsically nonreductive and its terms are defined in the same level of analysis in which the problem is stated. The descriptive approach has been the grand strategy of mathematical psychology—to represent the measurements obtained in behavioral experiments in a systematic and orderly form. That is, it is to match the course of an experimentally observed variable by means of one of the languages that can simulate or analogize the trajectories of empirical observations. To the extent that the theory follows that trajectory as well as the extent to which the theory predicts future events, a descriptive theory is considered to be a success.

In the past, largely because of the great variability of psychological findings, most descriptive theories of psychological function have been probabilistic or stochastic as opposed to deterministic in the manner so successfully used by the physical sciences.

> A descriptive theory is one that may track, or even predict, the trajectory of a set of observations, but does not reduce those representations to any lower level of analysis. Mathematical formulae, statistical averages, and verbal explanations are examples of descriptive theories as are simulations and behavioral observations.

The nature of descriptive theories is based on two considerations. Although the first is a matter of principled strategy (the neutrality of descriptions) the second is one driven by the practical empirical facts—there are still few solid empirical bridges from cognition to underlying neural structure.[10] The limited amount of neurophysiological thinking in modern mathematical psychology is clearly evidenced throughout its history. For example, consider the two volumes of the classic *Handbook of Mathematical Psychology* (Luce, Bush, & Galanter, 1963) in which neurophysiological language is almost completely limited to a single chapter on computer models and a few speculative neural-behavioral analogies. Examining current issues of the *Journal of Mathematical Psychology* shows that this trend continues.

Descriptive theories are not limited to psychology with its profound complexity and unresolved physiological foundations. It is not widely appreciated but even Newton's (1687) magnificent accomplishment *Principia Mathematica* was also a descriptive theory. He stated very explicitly in his eighth definition, "For I here design only to give a mathematical notion of those forces, without considering their physical causes or seats." This is a clear example of a descriptive, almost behavioral, albeit formal mathematical approach to science. It was left to other researchers to seek the physical "causes or seats" centuries later—a goal even now not yet fully achieved.

There is, of course, nothing intrinsically illicit or unsatisfactory about a descriptive theory; nonreductive physicalisms have been widely accepted by philosophers of science in which brains and minds are considered to be functions of the same kind of reality despite the fact that compelling epistemological barriers exist to prohibit direct communication between the two levels of discourse. Nonreductive (i.e., descriptive) theories have a long and fruitful history. However, I believe that cognitive neuroscience is special and demands more— ultimately a more complete neuroreductive theory—because its goal is specifically to explain cognition in neural terms. In this regard, it differs from many other sciences (e.g., conventional cognitive psychology) whose goals may be more patently descriptive. Whether we can approach such an ideal descriptive theory in cognitive neuroscience is yet to be determined.

Most psychological theories of cognitive activity, despite their complexity and formal mathematical structure, are descriptive only in the limited sense that they stimulate the invention of hypothetical constructs. That is, they are, for the most fundamental reasons, incapable of exclusively determining unique lower level mechanisms, by which I mean both cognitive and neurophysiological constructs. Similarly, control system models, such as those proposed by Powers (2005) also are purely descriptive. Although cloaked in the language of hardware control systems and functional processes such as "lag," "amplification," and "feedback," they are actually mathematical models of functions and processes that have no direct implications concerning what neurophysiological entities might implement those functions. Although there may be an element of analogy (that is, different behaviors may be modeled by the same level mathematics or statistics) between a steam engine and a human, there are not likely to be any material homologies. Even if there were, no descriptive model alone is capable of distinguishing between two alternative internal mechanisms, although it might predict the behavior of both quite well.

The point is that even the most formal, axiomatic, deductive, and accurately descriptive[11] mathematical theories are neutral concerning underlying mechanisms. The major reason for this constraint is straightforward: As previously noted, there are far too many plausible (as well as implausible) alternative neural mechanisms or hypothetical cognitive constructs that can produce the same behavior or experience, which is what we mean by "underdetermined." The information in a descriptive model is not sufficient to select a unique material instantiation from among these innumerable possible alternatives.

A modern, but still essentially descriptive analysis of psychological function, is typified by Luce's famous choice axiom and the theories that were stimulated by it. The choice axiom is a statement of behavior guiding the human propensity to make decisions from among a number of alternatives. Specifically, Luce (1959; 1977) proposed that if the choice of one object (A) was always preferred over another (B), then this preference order would remain the same no matter how many other items (C, D, E, etc.) were added to or deleted from the pool of objects.

The choice axiom is a fundamental postulate—that is, it is an axiomatic assumption (much like Newton's three laws) based on inductive reasoning from previous data (e.g., those collected by Clarke, 1957). It was assumed that this conjecture would hold robustly for other forms of choice behavior, that it would have generality, and, most important, that it could lead to other more complete, albeit still descriptive, theories of related forms of behavior. To the degree that this promise was fulfilled, the axiom could be confirmed and more comprehensive theories of human choice behavior derived. Over the years, by a combined process of confirming empirical evidence and mathematical derivations, this foundation axiom evolved into a general descriptive theory of choice behavior.

As a result of the empirical support for the choice axiom, it has been further developed into what has now become known as the Luce Choice Theory or as a Luce Process (Steele, 1974), both of which do creditable jobs of describing a variety of decision processes. The topics to which it has been applied include such diverse behaviors as handwriting, food preferences, estimates of the seriousness of crimes, and the order of lifted weights (See Luce, 1977, for a list of applications in which the choice axiom seems to hold.) More generally, theorems derived from the choice axiom have predicted human behavior in psychophysical tasks involved in scaling, recognition, detection, and discrimination (See Luce, 1963, for developments of this kind and the rest of the book edited by Luce et al., 1963, in which the Luce, 1963 axiom is applied to other behaviors.) Thus, the broad application of the axiom and the descriptive adequacy of the resulting theories have been confirmed.

The germane aspect of the development of Luce's derivations from the specific axiom to general theories in the present context is that the Luce choice axiom and the theories that derive from it are distinguished examples of nonreductive descriptions of cognitive activity typical of cognitive, psychological research. There are no allusions to anything neurophysiological throughout the literature of what many consider to be the most fully developed theory of cognitive activity. Although the theory may describe and predict, no matter how sophisticated and deductively coherent, it is completely neutral with regard to the neurophysiological mechanisms that might underlay the observed behavior. Although some investigators (e.g., Bundesen, Habekost, & Kyllingsbaek, 2005) have suggested bridging the essentially descriptive choice and reductive neural models, in fact, this can be done only by adding neurophysiological postulates to the theory, postulates that are actually totally separable from the behavioral components of the model and which have to be independently verified.

Like descriptive mathematical theories, the output of a computer simulation is underdetermined and, thus, there is no way that we can infer from its behavior alone how the underlying program produces the behavior it does. In other words, it is not possible to uniquely reverse engineer a system unless you have direct access to its components and their interactions.[12] Without auxiliary neurophysiological postulates, assumptions, and, most of all, relevant neurophysiological data, any descriptive program is fundamentally neutral with regard to underlying structure and mechanisms.

Why descriptive theories cannot be reductive is further accounted for by the fact they are confronted by the "many to one" constraint (Uttal, 2011). The "many to one" constraint is based on the fact that the information in a mathematical model (or, for that matter, any relevant behavioral data) is underdetermined; that is, insufficient information is available to determine which of a multitude of plausible and possible neural mechanisms (the many) might be producing the observed phenomenon (the one.)

Reductive Theories

By a reductive cognitive neuroscience theory, I refer to an approach to theoretical development in which an explicit effort is made to reduce cognition to some lower level of analysis, constructs, and mechanisms. For cognitive neuroscience, this target lower level is the neurophysiological one that can be populated by both macroneural and microneuronal mechanisms, entities, and functions. Purely psychological reductionist theories also exist and usually involve efforts to reduce behavior to "hypothetical constructs" (MacCorquodale & Meehl, 1948)—entities which are inferred but, unlike neurophysiological processes, cannot be directly observed. In general, I argue, if limited to these psychological level concepts and postulates and behavioral data, cognitive theories only can be descriptive and can be neither neurally or cognitively reductive for two main reasons—one conceptual and one empirical. First, they cannot be reduced to unique cognitive components or modules because there are innumerable possible combinations of such underlying mechanisms that can account for external behavior—the one to many constraint, again. In other words, behavior as well as all other indicators of mental activity are underdetermined with regard to its internal mechanisms. Second, they cannot be neurally reductive because the necessary neurophysiological knowledge that would support reductive theory is not available and may not ever be.

Despite the fact that neuroreductive theories attempt to link cognitive processes with neural mechanisms, few cognitive scientists concern themselves with the fundamental question of whether this kind of reduction is feasible. It is assumed, typically with little question or doubt, that a neuroreductive cognitive neuroscience theory will eventually exist based on the mass of neurophysiological findings.

> Reductive theories are those that invoke underlying mechanisms in their postulates and conclusions. In the context of cognitive neuroscience, this reduction is from behavior to neurophysiological mechanisms. However, psychology can also be reductive, for example, from behavior to cognitive modules.

I classify the special kind of reductive theory, the intellectual core of cognitive neurosciences, as "neuroreductive." Reductive theories are those that invoke, in addition to the function or process relations describing an activity, specific neurophysiological postulates about how underlying mechanisms might operate to account for those processes. They may or may not also have elaborate mathematical postulates, derivations, and theorems, but the unique attributes of a neuroreductive theory are that it includes specific statements about how functions of the nervous system are related to the behavior of interest. Indeed, it is the specific identities drawn between the neurophysiological and behavioral postulates that distinguish neuroreductive theories of cognitive processes from purely descriptive ones.

Unfortunately, many difficulties are encountered when attempts are made to develop a neuroreductive theory of a cognitive process or behavioral observation. There remains the practical difficulty of analyzing and evaluating the enormous complexity of the nervous system at any level of analysis. It is for this reason that most of the successful neuroreductive theories of cognitive processes are mainly carried out in the context of the most peripheral coding mechanisms of the sensory and motor systems where certain simplifying or regularizing (e.g., topological representation) constraints hold.

The classic and clearest example of competing neuroreductive theories of psychological processes and the attendant difficulties in resolving such controversies is embodied in the historical debate over the neural coding schemes of color experience. Prior to the second half of the 20th century, there was little neurophysiological information available to explain how visual wavelength information was encoded and transmitted to the central nervous system. At that time, it was hoped that visual theorists would be able to infer from the psychophysical data something about the nature of the underlying neural responses that transduced and conveyed "color" information; that is, the transmission codes.

The problem of inferring neural transmission codes from sensory experience was complicated by the unfortunate fact that there were two bodies of psychophysical (i.e., behavioral) data—opponent and trichromatic—that seemed relevant to the coding problem leading to opposite conclusions—the Young-Helmholtz trichromatic theory (invoked by Thomas Young, 1773–1829 and later by Hermann von Helmholtz, 1821–1894) and the Hering "opponent" colors theory proposed by Ewald Hering (1834–1918).

Young and Helmholtz argued that the resulting behavioral phenomenon must be due to having three kinds of color receptors in the eye. Hering, on the other hand, interpreted his data to mean that there was a biphasic, balanced, or opponent interaction between pairs of receptors in the retina. According to all of the then active color vision theorists, the psychophysical results were determined by alternative views of the response of the eye's receptor cells. It was, thus, a widely accepted scientific contention that one could make the logical leap from the psychophysical data to the neural mechanism. On the possibility of inference from function to structure, at least, they all agreed.[13]

All, however, made the same logical mistake by assuming that one can make unique inferences from psychophysical data to neural interpretations. Conversely, it can be argued that it is logically impossible for their respective neurophysiological theories to be substantiated by purely psychophysical data. This importance of this argument is supported by the persistence of the controversy; it lasted without resolution for over a century. What finally resolved the issue was the fact that the ascending visual pathways (including the retina) were simple enough for their neurophysiological inferences to be directly examined by recording from the individual cells of the retina—specifically the cone receptor and bipolar cells. Brown and Wald (1964) and Marks, Dobelle, and MacNichol (1964) demonstrated convincingly that the cones were trichromatic. The surprising result that followed was that, when the neuronal responses were measured by Tomita (1965) at the very next layer of the retina—the bipolar cells—these neurons turned out to be opponent-type in the sense proposed by Hering. Indeed, the codes used at higher levels of the visual system (e.g., by neurons in the lateral geniculate body of the thalamus) were subsequently shown by DeValois, Abramov, and Jacobs (1966) to display quite a different scheme than suggested by either the Young-Helmholtz or the Hering theories—some cells were opponent (both bi- and triphasic) and others were more like the monophasic responses of the trichromatic retinal receptors. Thus, different codes are being used at different stages in the visual pathway; but all are conveying the same information, just in different neural languages or codes.

What this bit of history suggests is manifold. First, it shows how different neurophysiological responses can be used at different levels of the nervous system to represent the same information. (This difficulty is exacerbated by the implication that there may be no single answer to any cognitive neuroscientific question because the system is not stable. From moment to moment and from subject to subject, a plethora of alternative representation schemes may be used.) Second, it illustrates the fundamental limitation on drawing inferences about the neuroanatomical substrates from behavioral or experiential data. Considering the difficulty in acquiring relevant and consistent neurophysiological data from the higher (i.e., cognitive) reaches of the central nervous system, it seems likely that few higher level cognitive processes are going to be resolved in the empirical manner that the sensory coding problem has been.

This historic episode, in retrospect, strongly argues that, with only certain very simple exceptions, the kind of inferences drawn from the peripheral sensory and motor systems in which unique structures are inferred from functional descriptions is not generally possible. I believe this inability to infer underlying neural structure from functional descriptions is a major flaw in both the philosophy and empirical approach of current cognitive neuroscience.

Top-Down and Bottom-Up Theories

We are reminded of another traditional dichotomy of different types of theories by Gerstner, Sprekeler, and Deco (2012). They divide theories into top-down and bottom-up categories. There is a vast difference between the two approaches. Bottom-up theories are generally based on relatively complete and concrete observations of the neurophysiology and neurochemistry of the microneuronal elements. The development of a putative theory of cognitive representation at this level of analysis is thus based on well-defined neurophysiological evidence, well-defined mathematical postulates, derivable deductive theorems, and compelling if not overwhelming data. However, this fine and complete level of neurophysiological detail is rarely an entrée into understanding cognitive process; it is much too low level (the entities of behavior and neurophysiology are still relatively poorly connected) and ignores the constraint imposed by the complex and idiosyncratic information processing interactions between huge numbers of neurons. Any hopes of a bottom-up theory of cognitive processes quickly drown in a sea of information despite the increasing availability of large-scale computers to simulate networks consisting of many neural components. The conceptual bridge between neural and psychological levels still remains uncrossed.

Top-down theories, in which we attempt to make inferential leaps from behavioral data to hypothetical neural mechanisms, are also seriously limited, but for quite different reasons than are bottom-up theories. I have repeatedly spoken of some of the difficulties involved in such an effort. Behavior, as well as mathematics, is fundamentally neutral with regard to underlying structure because so many alternatives are plausible but indistinguishable. Further complicating the top-down approach is the fact that much of the required neural information on which such a theory must be based is lost in the cumulative signals exemplified by macroneural measures such as the fMRI.

What happens in this case is that top-down and bottom-up theories tend to evolve in quite different directions. Bottom-up theories tend to be relatively constrained, for example, the Hodgkin and Huxley (1952) model, which went from well-developed ideas of ions and their concentrations to the responses of individual neuronal responses. Top-down theories, on the other hand, typified by molar behavior and cumulative macroneural responses, tend to infer from high-level responses to underlying "constructs" and "intuitions" as well as "neurophysiological operators" that have actually left no deductive trail. Whether it will be possible for top-down and bottom-up theories to converge on a unified explanatory theory is yet to be determined.

As a result, pure top-down theories tend to be unconstrained "simulations" in which the underlying processes are plausible and possible rather than based on robust and relevant empirical observations. As Gerstner et al. (2012) pointed out, "It is difficult to control a complex simulation if we do not have an intuition of the basic mechanisms at work" (p. 64) and those necessary intuitions are generally not available to the behaviorist. The situation is the reverse for bottom-up theories; they typically have solid concepts of what constitute the constituent component mechanisms but cannot bridge the gap between brain and mind.

Bottom-up theories, therefore, fail easily although they may initially be successful (the possibility of falsification is an advantage according to Popper, 1963) in the light of discrepant predictions. Top-down theories, on the other hand, are, unfortunately, much more resilient because the inferred lower level entities on which they are founded can be easily adjusted by modifying equations or constructs to make the theory fit. Thus, top-down theories tend to be simulations using whatever inferred entities and processes can be conscripted or invented to make the simulation work. A cryptic disadvantage of top-down simulations, therefore, is that they can be easily tweaked and tuned to fit data by invoking or modifying whatever extra concepts or computational tools are needed to fit the observations.

1.5 What Is a Full or Complete Theory?

The complexity of the linguistic issues that must be clarified to understand the role of theory in cognitive neuroscience is substantial. Frequently used terms such as "explanation," "prediction," "sufficiency," and "necessity" are bandied about in sometimes ambiguous contexts. To understand what would constitute a full and complete theory, it is necessary to examine what some of these words mean. In the following section, I consider a few of these problematic terms and point out why they contribute to the difficulties of developing really robust theories.

A particularly salient word lurking in the background of any discussion of theory is "explanation." In some basic sense, explanation and its near synonyms such as "understanding" and "rationalization" (as well as less ambitious terms as "accounts for") are the ultimate goals of theoretical science. Theories, in this context, are the specific instantiations of the more general term "explanation." A multitude of scholars in the last few decades have wrestled with the complexities of explanation in science in general (e.g., Hempel, 1965; Nagel, 1979) as well as in psychology in particular (e.g., Cummins, 1983). Most raise questions more than provide answers to the question of what is a theory or an explanation and how complete can it be.

In cognitive neuroscience, by definition, only reductive theories can aspire to be complete explanations; descriptive ones are, by definition, incomplete in that they are not constructed from the known lower level machinery of neural responses. A complete reductive theory would provide relevant reductive answers to all of the salient questions concerning the causes and mechanisms of some phenomenon. A common confusion is between prediction and description, on the one hand, and complete reductive explanation, on the other. Although some philosophers and many cognitive neuroscientists equate the two, prediction does not necessarily incorporate all of the details required of a complete explanation. Formal, descriptive, mathematical theories may predict with complete accuracy the trajectory of a phenomenon by tracing past behavior; however, it may do so without any understanding of the underlying neural mechanics, processes, and operations of that phenomenon. Indeed, this is what Newton meant by saying that he deals with the forces "without considering their physical causes or seats." This is also the modus operandi of modern psychological theorizing. Psychological theorists describe behavior and infer plausible cognitive "modules" that might account for the observed phenomena. By definition, psychological theories are neither unique nor neuroreductive no matter how well they may predict behavior. Complete explanation requires more than prediction; the one is not the same as the other. A probabilistic description of a phenomenon can produce highly accurate estimates of the likelihood that a particular measurement will occur in time, space, or magnitude but offers little in the way of explanation of the actual neural mechanisms underlying that phenomenon.

Practical considerations raise serious questions about the difficulty and even possibility of providing full neural explanations of any cognitive process. For these and many other reasons, fully reductive explanations (and, thus, totally comprehensive and overarching theories) may possibly be conceived only in some ideal sense. The abstract ideal of a complete explanation of the mind-brain problem is increasingly appreciated to be an enormously difficult issue that has become an epistemological topic in its own right. What would constitute a full neuroreductive explanation of some cognitive phenomenon? Obviously, in complex systems like the mind-brain, it is not going to be an easy task to answer this question, and it may have many different components. One of the most interesting and comprehensive approaches to providing a full theoretical explanation is the 2,500-year-old scheme originally expressed by Aristotle (384 BC–322 BC) and brought to modern prominence once again by Killeen (2001). Aristotle, according to Killeen, referred to four "causes" or kinds of explanation: Material, formal, final, and efficient. To a first approximation, a complete theory of anything would entail precise statements of each of these respective four causes.

The Aristotelian four causes are really the partial modes of theoretical explanation that seek to answer four related questions for many different sciences.

For cognitive neurosciences and psychology, these four questions are as follows:

- Material causes ask, what are the neural mechanisms underlying some behavior and how do they interact? This is the goal of modern cognitive neuroscience.
- Formal causes ask, how can we describe the activity patterns of a system using a statistical, mathematical, or even a mechanical model simulating cognitive processes? This is the goal of modern mathematical psychology.
- Final causes ask, what is the purpose of some mechanism? This should be a forbidden zone in modern scientific psychology because it suggests a teleology—an a priori anticipated and purposeful target as opposed to an eventual purpose being determined by random variation. Asked in reverse— what kind of mechanism could account for some function, it becomes very familiar—the fallacious proclivity of many psychologists to infer structure from function. Because of the inaccessibility of the mechanisms underlying a behavior and their basic underdetermined nature, this is, in most cases, probably an unanswerable question. Nevertheless, this is the goal of evolutionary psychology.
- Efficient causes ask, what is the trigger stimulus for a particular behavior? This is the role of modern behaviorism: Manipulate the stimuli, measure the responses, and, if possible, infer possible functional transformations between the two. Experimental psychologists have operated under this umbrella behaviorist paradigm for many years regardless of their professed commitment to a modular Cognitive Psychology.[14]

The Aristotelian four causes are presented as an example of the necessary components of a "complete" theoretical explanation of some phenomenon. To Aristotle, a theory is full and complete to the degree that it provides answers to all four causes. However elegant such an idea may be, achieving the goal for cognitive neuroscience remains elusive simply because in some cases the four causes can be internally contradictory and, for practical reasons, can only rarely simultaneously be determined. In cognitive psychology, developing formal and efficient causes is what one tends to do when material and final causes of a phenomenon cannot be determined.

The material cause, of course, is of the greatest interest to cognitive neuroscientists. It is also the most difficult to achieve—a factor to which current activity in this field attests. According to one group of investigators (Martin, Grimwood, & Morris, 2000), confirming that a particular neural mechanism is the underlying mechanism of a particular cognitive process would require manipulations of the nervous system that are far beyond any conceivable technology.

In this book, I use the word theory in a very specific context. For my purposes, a "full and complete" neuroreductionist theory is the ultimate explanation of the manner in which mind emerges from brain as explained in terms of the neurophysiology of the brain. Unfortunately, the complexity of the mind-brain system is such that the search for such an overarching theory may be an unobtainable quest.

There are, of course, valid reasons to define "theory" in different terms and with different meanings. For example, Killeen (2012, personal communication) invokes the term to denote "symbol systems that communicate important facts about data." To him, a theory is primarily a mapping of data; its success depends mainly upon the success of the symbol system (i.e., the theory) to describe observations in a practical way. This is, of course, a much less ambitious goal than the search for a "full and complete" theory. It is more comparable to description than to neuroreductive explanation in the strong neuroreductionist sense I emphasize here. For me, the holy grail of a full and complete theory is far more demanding than Killeen's "symbol system." It involves understanding of the properties of the components of a lower level of mechanisms, their interactions, and the manner in which their functions are transmuted into cognitive processes. It depends on the integration of lower level observations to reproduce higher level properties. A solely descriptive mapping of higher level properties (i.e., behavior) is insufficient to serve as a substitute for the ultimate kind of theory hoped for by cognitive neuroscientists in their efforts to solve the mind-brain problem.

1.6   Interim Summary

This chapter has introduced the general idea of theory as it is expressed in the context of modern cognitive neuroscience. Perhaps the most salient conclusion to which one can come after reading a lot of this kind of research publication is that the word "theory" is ambiguously used by investigators in this field. It is in the ideal sense of a pyramiding of specific findings into general rules that the word approaches a specific definition, if not actualization. Surprisingly, one of the most complete and cogent specifications of what is a "theory" remains Aristotle's four causes. Unfortunately, identifying all four causes is an outcome that is rare to the point of nonexistence.

Two main types of theories must also be distinguished. Descriptive theories merely chart the course of a process but the data on which they are based are underdetermined and cannot by themselves uniquely identify underlying mechanisms. Reductive theories attempt to go a step further by identifying what the underlying mechanisms of a process may be. Reductive theories may be either neuroreductively (to neural components) or cognitively (to cognitive modules) reductive.

The near aim of this book is to evaluate the status of the macroneural approach to cognitive neuroscience theory in the second decade of the 21st century. It is not yet certain that a full and complete macroneural mind-brain theory is obtainable; the losses of salient information when measurements are made at the macroneural level argue against success in the short run.

Other fundamental factors to be discussed here raise the possibility, at least, that no full and complete reductive theory is possible. This is a very important issue because large investments are being made under the assumption that an overarching theory may someday be possible and even larger ones have been promised by our government for the future. Unfortunately, the philosophers may have had it right in that the mind-brain problem may be intractable, a conclusion much to the distaste of cognitive neuroscientists.

The remainder of this book looks mainly at the current state of what constitutes macroreductive theory of higher cognitive processes. Chapter 2 presents a discussion of the varieties of theories that now appear in the literature, an initial attempt to categorize them, and a critique of some attempts to prematurely create new interdisciplinary cognitive neurosciences. Chapter 3 deals with some important conceptual issues in the field and introduces us to the main prevailing connectionist theory. Chapter 4 considers the current status, goals, and limits of macroneural connectionist theory. Chapter 5 examines the limitations of connectionist theory. There, I identify the influences that gave rise to them as well as those that will define their future. Finally, Chapter 6 draws out some of the implications and emerging principles that are becoming clear in recent years.

Notes

1. This introductory section is an abbreviated and updated version of a much more extensive discussion presented in Uttal (2005) introducing the concept of theory. Any of my readers who would like to delve deeper into this topic are directed there and to the references cited there. Older ideas expressed there are reinterpreted in the context of new ideas in this new work.

2. It is in definitions like these that the confusions of a limited hypothesis or conjecture with a full-blown theory are made explicit.

3. Of course, simple correlation is not sufficient to serve as a theoretical explanation. Correlations can exist for many reasons without implying any causation. For example, it is possible to find correlations between fMRI signals and cognitive processes that are not due to any brain-mind factors but might be due to some intervening third factor. A basic question that must be asked: What kind of questions can be asked and then answered with each of these methodologies?

4. Although it has popular for several years to point out the "seductive" influence of brain images (McCabe & Castel, 2008; Weisberg et al., 2008), Farah and Hook (2013) now argue that there is increasing evidence that this allure is a myth. However, their critique is based on experiments that were carried out 5 years apart. A real "seductive influence" of brain images then may have been explained by their relative novelty. Subjects in the recent experiments who do not show the effect may simply have changed in the intervening years, having become much more sophisticated. Thus, both sets of experiments, although seemingly contradictory, may be correct.

5. After five editions, the standard diagnostic tool for mental processes—the *Diagnostic and Statistical Manual of Mental Disorders (DSM)*—remains an extremely controversial book filled with indistinguishable illnesses with different names or single illnesses with multiple names. The *DSM* does not deal with biomarkers per se but rather is a set of descriptions of abnormal behaviors. It also has the defect of not being stable; behavior classified as abnormal in one generation is accepted as normal in another mirroring popular and political culture, rather than real pathologies. Recently it has been rejected by the Director of the National Institute of Mental Health as a set of criteria for research support.

6. One exception to this generalization was my earlier book *A Taxonomy of Visual Processes* (Uttal, 1981), which dealt with a narrow range of visual topics.

7. Psychology's traditional .05 threshold (equivalent to about 2 standard deviations) for significance can be compared with the criterion used in particle physics—.0000006 (equivalent to about 5 standard deviations—a very conservative criterion used in the seemingly successful search for the Higgs boson). Even given the differences between the subject matters, there is the suggestion that psychology's .05 is far too lenient. Cognitive neuroscientists often use $p = .001$, which is better but still subject to interpretive error.

8. It goes without further comment that any theory worthy of its name must be empirically reliable and testable. This admonition operates at all levels of scientific inquiry, not just at the pinnacle of synoptic theory. Establishing the validity and reliability of our observations is the primary role played by experimentation. In addition, it must be logically plausible. Establishing plausibility is the role played by logic and mathematics.

9. A similar dichotomy of description and reduction has been used by Wittgenstein (1958) in characterizing the types of explanations available to philosophers. He argued that for philosophy "It can never be our job to reduce anything to anything or to explain anything. Philosophy is purely descriptive" (p. 18). However, it can be argued that, in principle, cognitive neuroscience can aspire to explanation and reduction because it has available both descriptive and reductive information from several levels of analysis, whereas philosophy is essentially stuck at the same level as are purely behavioral observations—descriptions.

10. This may seem like an overstatement when one considers the amount of activity in the field of current cognitive neuroscience. I refer my readers to several of my earlier books that make this argument more completely than I have here.

11. By "accurately descriptive," I mean that the mathematical expressions follow and predict the trajectory of a cognitive process with accuracy. Unfortunately, as discussed earlier, all such formal descriptions are neutral with regard to underlying mechanisms; there are innumerable cognitive or neural (or both) mechanisms that can produce the same trajectory. Unless one adds specific neurophysiological postulates to a descriptive "theory," there is no way to challenge such a theory to reveal its possible underlying mechanisms.

12. This kind of reverse engineering is analogous to that kind rejected by Poldrack (2006). He admonishes cognitive neuroscientists against inferring a particular cognitive process from "the activation of a particular brain region" (p. 59). Because brain activations in a particular place may be involved in any number of cognitive activities and are, therefore, "not deductively valid" (p. 59), they, like behavior and other functional processes, are undetermined as implied by Poldrack. What he offers as a partial

solution is the use of a Bayesian analysis in which prior information is introduced into the analysis. However, his criticism is clear: The usefulness of "imperfect" reverse inference is limited.

13. There is an assumption in both of these theories that has a number of implications. It is that the specific nature of the receptor's function is the "cause" or "mechanism" of the experience. This assumption ignores the possibility that alternative codes could produce the same response. This issue also concerns the codes used at higher levels of the ascending visual pathway—would they necessarily have to be the same, or are different codes possible at each stage of processing? If so, what then does the psycho-physical data mean neurophysiologically? I argue that the answer to this rhetorical question is—nothing. Overall system behavior cannot definitively distinguish between alternative internal neural mechanisms.

14. Cognitive psychology is the main theme of modern experimental psychology. It is characterized by an effort to define and determine the basic thought processes under-lying behavior and the assumption that such a goal is achievable. It emerged in the middle of the 20th century as a reaction to behaviorism, which in its most extreme forms largely ignored the information processing steps between the stimuli and the responses. Serious questions remain about the achievability of this kind of cognitive reductionism. From the point of view of many of us, this hope motivated genera-tions of experimental psychologists to deny what is a more realistic and modest science of behaviorist psychology.

2

PROTOTHEORIES AND NONTHEORIES

2.1 Introduction

In Chapter 1, I introduced the general concept of a theory and pointed out the ambiguities regarding the variety of meanings of this well-used word. In addition, I specified what the word "theory" meant to me in the context of this present book. I also introduced a mini-taxonomy of the types of nontheories, prototheories, and complete theories that have so far been offered up to organize, describe, explain, and summarize empirical data concerning the relation between the mind and the brain. In this chapter, I examine specific examples of cognitive neuroscience "theories" that do not meet my criteria for designation as anything other than a prototheory. This task is made difficult by the fact that the brain image approaches to cognitive neuroscience are still quite young. Despite a substantial corpus of published empirical articles, research in this field is still dominated by the search for empirical correlations and localizations rather than syntheses.

Furthermore, categorizing existing theories is much more arbitrary than it may at first seem for a number of reasons. Among the most obvious difficulty is the fact that the required empirical foundation for theory building is still in an underdeveloped state in cognitive neuroscience—most of us are still struggling to develop methods and obtain empirical results about the basic nature of brain organization and representation. Comprehensive and accurate theories extrapolating from specific experiments to general laws are still relatively underdeveloped compared with the physical sciences. It is not yet certain whether this is a fundamental intractability or just the birth pangs of a new science.

Furthermore, despite the huge corpus of empirical research published in this field, there is still a paucity of reliable results on which to build synthetic or synoptic theories. If the ideal goal of a theory is to integrate data and abstract general principles, there is an a priori requirement that the empirical foundation be sufficiently robust, repeatable, and consistent that whatever general principles are being expressed should actually be represented by these data. The reliability question is fundamental and yet has not received the attention that it deserves in a world of ambiguous stimuli and highly complex, multicellular organ systems such as the brain. Indeed, the issue has only recently been raised in a series of articles in *Science* for a variety of other, arguably simpler, sciences. Peng (2011), for example, discusses the problem for computational science; Tomasello and Call (2011) for primate cognition; Ryan (2011) for field biology; Ioannidis and Khoury (2011) for genetics; and Santer, Wigley, and Taylor (2011) for atmospheric temperatures. Surprisingly, the field of cognitive neuroscience, the domain of what some of us consider to be less reliable data, was not mentioned.

Another problem inhibiting theoretical progress in cognitive neuroscience is the uncertain and often vague way in which cognitive phenomena are defined in psychological research. It is not always clear what tasks or stimuli are being studied when a particular term is used to describe them. For example, the term "working memory" can represent a wide variety of different experimental protocols because of slight differences in methodology, uncontrolled properties of the independent variable, or the intent of the investigator.

Thus, if one seeks to find reliable equivalences or correlations, much less causal relations between cognitive phenomena and neural responses, it demands an increased degree of precision in the definition of the key stimulus variables in an experiment. Unfortunately, different investigators use different terminologies to specify what is often the same cognitive process. One researcher's search for data backing up a theory of decision making, for example, may be operationally indistinguishable from another's effort to study attention. This is the inverse of the additional problem in which the same words may be used to define what may operationally be very different cognitive processes.

Therefore, we have to take it as a given that cognitive neuroscience is profoundly influenced by the vagueness of psychological language. Clarifying psychological definitions and constructs should also be a high-priority task for this science especially. Nevertheless, this important task is largely ignored by all but a few psychologists and cognitive neuroscientists. Currently, psychological terms are defined largely by the operations involved in carrying out an experiment. This can lead to serious confusions of definition, as exemplified by the work of Vimal (2009) who tabulated 40 different definitions of the term "consciousness." In Uttal (2011), I also was able to identify an equal number of terms that designated some form of learning.

Furthermore, the exact relation between a cognitive process and a neural response is not always clear even in the most highly correlated data. It is, for example, not clear what the oft-used term "accounts for" means. Yet this is a commonly used phrase by cognitive neuroscientists. "Accounts for" could have any of the following meanings:

- Statistical correlation between cognitive and neural responses
- A functionally unrelated indicator in the sense of a "biomarker"
- The location of a neural mechanism of a cognitive process
- The psychoneural equivalent of a cognitive process[1]

> The psychoneural equivalent is the actual neural mechanism some of whose activities are indistinguishable from the cognitive process itself. In other words, the psychoneural equivalent *is* the cognitive process. Although defined in different languages (cognition and neurophysiology), the different words may denote exactly the same thing. Determining the nature of the psychoneural equivalent is an extremely challenging task facing many impediments and obstacles but is the holy grail of cognitive neuroscience.

It is also true that our prototheories and theories are strongly, if not overwhelmingly, influenced by our contemporary technology. Modern brain imaging instrumentation forces us to ask the question of mind-brain relationships in a particular way—where are the part or the parts of the brain that are maximally responsive during a given cognitive process?[2] Whether any answer to such a question is sufficient to identify the psychoneural equivalent is uncertain. The imaging technology drives what kind of data we can obtain and the data ultimately determine what kind of theory can be generated. In the domain of functional brain imaging, because the kind of data obtained is restricted to the macroneural location and arrangement of broad regions of the brain, it is not possible to delve deeply into the microneuronal features of the great neuronal networks.

Yet it is at the level of the collective but unpooled state of the neuronal networks (not that of either individual neurons or of the cumulative fMRI signals) that the critical information processing mechanisms are thought by most cognitive neuroscientists to most likely reside. There are, however, formidable combinatorial barriers of numerousness and complexity blocking analysis at this level. According to Koch (2012), the combinatorial complexity of a relatively simple real neuronal network (e.g., the two million neurons of the visual cortex of a mouse) would take about 10 million years to "fully characterize" even with the most optimistic view of what computers might be in the future. This situation would be partially ameliorated, he further noted, if the brain could be clumped into functional modules, but it would still take 6 years under the best of conditions and with the most powerful of computers to carry out the necessary computations. Koch concluded, however,

"For if appropriate modules cannot be found, understanding of life will escape us" (p. 532). This assertion highlights the dreadful effect that brain complexity could have on cognitive neuroscience: We may never be able to answer some of the most profound questions of human existence, although we learn much and cure many.

There are other restrictions imposed by several factors on the inferences that can be drawn from brain imaging data in particular. First, the boundaries between brain regions are anatomically ill-defined. Second, responses cannot be localized to the level of microneuronal neuronal networks because of their limited spatial resolution. Therefore, their resolution, although improving all the time, is not yet fine enough to study the activity of networks of individual neurons. Third, much of the relevant information describing neuronal activity at the microneuronal level is lost by the biological, instrumental, and statistical pooling processes that combine and merge the cellular electrophysiological responses into an inseparable amalgamation.

Given these constraints, the primary questions that are answerable with brain imaging techniques are variations on the theme of spatial localization; that is, *where* are the parts of the brain that are concomitantly activated with particular cognitive processes and how are they interconnected? Despite this limitation, this question is often approached from a number of different points of view, each with subtly different connotations. Although these differing connotations will become evident as I review the various kinds of research carried out to attack the problem of mind-brain relations at this macroneural level of analysis, it is useful at this point to tabulate some of the issues that have been considered by investigators using brain imaging devices in their search for the foundations of a mind-brain theory at this level.

1. As noted, the prototypical question asked by investigators using brain imaging techniques is, *where* are the parts of the brain that become active when a particular cognitive process is underway?

2. Another level of inquiry is how, both in general and specific terms, are the salient brain areas interconnected at the macroneural level for cognitive operations? This was initially conceptualized as an *anatomic* question dealing with the nature of the interconnections (mediated by white, in other words, myelinated bands of axons) between regions. However, there is a functional analog that has generated much current interest—how are the parts of the brain *functionally* interconnected when particular cognitive processes are being carried out? Theories of this kind require much more elaborate analytic algorithms than simple tabulation of activated regions. However, they are really just another version of answers to the basic "where" question; one generalized to systems of interacting nodes rather than unique function-specific locations. The ultimate goal of this approach is to determine the connectivity

among brain regions during cognition and then describe the properties of the resulting networks.

3. Classic physiological psychology has traditionally been aimed as associating anatomic brain mechanisms with particular cognitive processes by extirpative, stimulating, or recording techniques. However, in large part those kinds of research are beset by ill-defined and invasive surgical procedures and preexisting assumptions about regional functions and, in large part have currently been replaced by imaging techniques. Traditional work done using lesioning as the main tool (e.g., Kennard, 1955) has been much reduced, to be replaced mainly by fMRI techniques.

4. A classic problem that seemingly has been empirically resolved in the favor of distributed responses was the debate between those who argued that the brain correlates of cognitive processes were well-localized and function-specific regions, on the one hand, and those who felt that the responses were distributed over broad multifunctional regions of the brain, on the other. The accumulating scientific evidence seems to increasingly support the latter conclusion. However, the details of this debate remain controversial, attracting the attention of a number of investigators.

5. Cognitive scientists have proposed that current research with brain images will be able to resolve some purely psychological controversies. The question is, can neurophysiology inform psychology? This is a form of hypothesis testing that depends on testable neurophysiological postulates being included within what are otherwise purely psychological theories. The debate over the applicability of brain imaging data to theory building rages on. (See the discussion between Coltheart, 2006, an opponent of the idea that any psychological theory controversy has *yet* been resolved by brain imaging techniques, and Henson, 2006, who believed that they have.)

6. A major long-term and highly controversial issue in brain imaging cognitive neuroscience is, can these techniques be used to read the mind; in other words, to tell us what a person was thinking about or perceiving by examining the fMRI data? Although there has been some progress in selecting alternate sensory responses from among a limited set of brain images, much of this modest achievement seems to be attributable to topologically preserved peripheral sensory encoding. For example, visual stimuli are represented by retinotopic maps in the primary sensory area that preserve the topology of stimuli and, thus, may maintain accessible and useful information about the spatial pattern of a stimulus. This is not possible with the symbolic brain representations driven by higher order cognitive processes that have no isomorphic relations between brain activity and those cognitive processes.

7. Many cognitive neuroscientists, heavily informed by psychological taxonomies, are trying to use brain imaging devices to determine something about

the localized brain mechanisms by which cognitive processes are carried out. For example, how do we learn? What brain changes occur in learning? A major unsolved problem is where and what is the engram—the actual storage medium of memory? Many seek to understand the emergence of consciousness, attention, and other vaguely defined high-level cognitive processes by determining which brain regions are activated when these cognitive processes are manipulated. This is the main theme of much of brain imaging research these days. However, there are strong reasons to believe that this simplistic concept of seeking correspondences between cognitive processes and brain locations may be ill-chosen.

8. A specific, unresolved question is the relation between the macroneural brain images and the microneuronal neuronal responses. We assume that the former is the summation of the latter but there are few definitive statements of their relationship. Some have associated fMRI signals with spike activity (Smith et al., 2002), whereas others have suggested that their origins are to be found in local potentials (Ekstrom, 2010).

9. There are many technical issues that occupy the time and energies of cognitive scientists, not all of which are aimed at the great question of how the mind emerges from brain processes. There is a continued effort to develop techniques to extract the best possible and largest amount of data from noisy brain images. Still other investigators are concerned with the technical matter of how we can pool or combine methods with low statistical power to produce higher power experiments in order to produce more significant data. Depending on what are the actual signal-to-noise relations and whether a signal actually exists or is a manifestation of a stochastic system, this may also be an ill-chosen expenditure of resources.

10. Most generally, cognitive neuroscience is aimed at establishing the neural (or neuronal) basis of cognition. In short, the main goal of this science is to provide some insights into the great question, how does the brain make the mind? To this overarching question, there is little in the way of either an answer or a satisfactory theory yet available. It is highly problematic if we have even begun to answer this question given the likelihood that macroneural techniques like the fMRI may actually obscure the critical microneuronal information that would answer this question.

Obviously, whereas some of these questions and goals represent issues that are of existential importance, others are of less ontological significance. Equally obviously, not all of the cognitive neuroscience questions posed here are currently answerable. For those that can be answered, some of the answers will emerge from prototheories discussed in this and subsequent chapters.

In the following sections, I present specific examples of nontheories and prototheories of how the brain represents or encodes cognitive processes.

2.2 Nontheories—Is Localization a Foundation for Theory?

The brain imaging approach to cognitive neuroscience is a relatively new way of studying the mind-brain relationship; at best, it is little more than two decades old. In general, its goal is to determine which regions are consistently associated with particular cognitive processes. In many, if not most, such explorations, the answer to this most basic question is still uncertain. Indeed, it is not even certain that the basic question of localization is a good one; it is possible that the concept of associating macroneural brain areas and cognitive process is a misdirection that diverts us from achieving an understanding of the actual mind-brain relationship.

The conceptual postulate, therefore, that dominates current cognitive neuroscience research is what we might refer to as the "traditional localization" concept. Essentially, this type of research is "barefoot" empirical but not directly theoretical; it is but a preliminary step in the acquisition of data that might help to build more comprehensive theories in the future. "Successful" experiments are those that are able to consistently associate particular localized peaks of regional activations with particular stimulus or task conditions. To the degree that these associations are robust, investigators are limited to identifying and tabulating them.[3]

There prevails a highly questionable assumption guiding the research protocols in this particular mode of attack on the mind-brain problem. That is, that the inferred modular components of a cognitive process will map in some repeatable and neurophysiologically coherent way onto localized regions of the brain. As widely accepted as this hypothesis is, there have been persistent logical reasons and are now an increasing number of empirical reasons to question it. The psychological processes and phenomena for which localized representations are assumed to exist are not necessarily dimensionally isomorphic with the brain's natural spatial layout. The cognitive processes are, it must also be remembered, themselves typically the instantiation of our experimental designs and not necessarily of any simple property of functional behavior. Whether they are divisible into the "hypothetical constructs" or intervening "modules or faculties" that correspond to specific anatomical regions or structures of the brain is uncertain.

The implications and inferences of hypotheses and theories must then be empirically tested to determine if they continue to hold more generally. However easy to put this essential step of the process into words, it is not that simple to execute. Indeed, it is conversely true that when you are dealing with a system whose stimuli are at least multifactorial and for which the exact triggering stimuli are obscure, whose responses are multidimensional and redundant, and for which there may be no direct relation of the stimulus to cognitive response, the probability of finding any kind of a response that satisfies the a priori theoretical judgments of investigators becomes artificially and incorrectly enhanced.

One sound recent report of a traditional "localization" experiment exemplifying this protocol was reported by Farrow et al. (2011). They were interested in the ability of their subjects to perceive social hierarchies. Their goal was to determine the brain regions that were involved in this cognitive process. They asked their subjects in a way that required forced-choice answers to questions such as, which of two pictures indicated someone higher in the social hierarchy? From their experimental results, they concluded:

> Both social hierarchy and social alliance judgments activated left ventrolateral prefrontal cortex (VLPFC), left dorsal inferior frontal gyrus (IFG) and bilateral fusiform gyri. In addition, social alliance judgments activated right dorsal IFG and medial prefrontal cortex. When compared directly with social alliance, social hierarchy judgments activated left orbitofrontal cortex. Detecting the presence of social hierarchies and judging other's relative standing within them implicates the cognitive executive, in particular the VLPFC.
>
> *(p. 1552)*

Thus, this study was a purely empirical approach characteristic of much of the current work in the field embodying what I have referred to as a "traditional approach." I do not mean this as a pejorative criticism; obviously this kind of research is a necessary antecedent to subsequent theory building, and this work seems to be a well thought out and clear example of this fundamental empirical approach of much of the research in this field. However, does it represent a prototheory of the mind-brain relation? I personally feel that research of this kind is only collecting empirical facts and that their conclusions, like a host of other similar studies, do not represent even the glimmerings of a prototheory. The facts have accumulated, but the consolidation of those facts into a theory or even prototheory has not yet occurred.

Farrow and his colleagues were not alone in their essentially pretheoretical, empirical approach. Nor do they claim to be in search of a theory. Most other current brain imaging researchers seem to have this same limited goal, as evidenced by the conclusions each draws from their experimental studies. Samples of similar research conclusions are now presented:[4]

- The results support distinct dorsal-ventral locations for phonological and semantic processes within the LIFG [Left Inferior Frontal Gyrus]. (Costafreda et al., 2006, p. 799)
- Taken together, our meta-analysis reveals that animals and tools are categorically represented in visual areas but show convergence in higher-order associative areas in the temporal and frontal lobes in regions that are typically regarded as being involved in memory and/or semantic processing. Our results also reveal that naming tools not only engages visual areas in the ventral stream but also a fronto-parietal network associated with tool use. (Chouinard & Goodale, 2010, p. 409)

- In this review of 100 fMRI studies of speech comprehension and production, published in 2009, activation is reported for prelexical speech perception in bilateral superior temporal gyri; meaningful speech in middle and inferior temporal cortex; semantic retrieval in the left angular gyrus and pars orbitalis; and sentence comprehension in bilateral superior temporal sulci. For incomprehensible sentences, activation increases in four inferior frontal regions, posterior planum temporale, and ventral supramarginal gyrus. These effects are associated with the use of prior knowledge of semantic associations, word sequences, and articulation that predict the content of the sentence. Speech production activates the same set of regions as speech comprehension. In addition, activation is reported for word retrieval in left middle frontal cortex; articulatory planning in the left anterior insula; the initiation and execution of speech in left putamen, pre-SMA, SMA, and motor cortex; and for suppressing unintended responses in the anterior cingulate and bilateral head of caudate nuclei. (Price, 2010, p. 62)

The point is that all of these studies were investigating the straightforward problem of brain localization of cognitive processes in an empirical manner that is hard pressed even to be called a prototheory.

Whatever the outcome of this kind of research that seeks to answer the "where" question, such studies do little to either explicate interpretations or inform theories beyond tabulating regional and cognitive co-occurrences. They represent empirical results that have not yet, but may sometime, be integrated into a theory. Nor, I suspect, was achieving the goal of developing theory the intent of any of these investigators. I present them here as examples of the kind of essentially explorative work on the localization of cognitive-related processes that has dominated much of brain imaging research by cognitive neuroscientists in the past two decades—they are truly "data without theories."

Others might well differ with this point of view by emphasizing that these findings are themselves harbinger of a theory or at least a prototheory. To the degree that such a statement is supported by robust empirical findings, this argument gains considerable force. There is nothing beyond the raw findings offered by these conclusions; there are rarely inferences that go beyond the data nor are there either descriptions or reductive explanations that extend our understanding beyond the bare bones of the data themselves. They are more analogous to the preliminary explorative stages of other sciences. Others will subsequently have to carry out the synthetic process to integrate these findings into what we mean by a comprehensive or overarching theory.

2.3 Nontheories—Data Extraction, Accumulation, and Analysis Techniques

Simple recapitulations of the data obtained during a brain-imaging study are not the only kind of nontheoretical data that have proliferated in cognitive neuroscience. Often cryptically confused with reductive or descriptive theories of the mind-brain problem are the complex analytical techniques that are used to extract data from noisy background situations. The basic reason for this confusion is the fact that the fMRI signal-to-noise ratios in brain image responses are often too low for the salient data to be easily extracted without powerful analytic manipulations from the "random" background fluctuations influencing the experiment.

As impressive as some of the modern analyses of brain imaging data may be, it is important to appreciate that much of this analytic effort to extract data is actually secondary to the psychobiological task at hand. Their role is to extract and quantify salient data from the background noise that character-izes this kind of research. Cognitive science's theoretical goal is to link these extracted neural data to cognitive phenomena in as reductive a manner as possible. It is, therefore, essential that the differences between data analysis techniques, on the one hand, and reductive cognitive neuroscience theories, on the other, be kept in mind. Although the ultimate goal for cognitive neuroscientists is to explain mind-brain relationships, and although these data analysis techniques are a necessary preliminary step to assure that the data on which cognitive neuroscience theories are based are valid, they are neither descriptive or reductive theories.

In sum, with few exceptions, the field of cognitive neuroscience is currently at the preliminary stage of exploration that every science must go through. There are some pioneering formal theories (see Chapter 4) that describe the resulting data, but these are largely descriptive and not reductive. There is still no answer to the general question of how the brain makes the mind, and an increasingly compelling suggestion that the brain imaging approach may never go beyond that descriptive stage. It is clear that brain imaging explorations seeking cogni-tively significant correlations with localized brain regions are limited to identifying the regions of the brain at which concurrent activity is generated by what are often ill-defined cognitive tasks. However, tabulation of these areas does not constitute a "theory" in the integrative sense defined earlier.

The next sections of this chapter deal with some data analysis techniques that have the proclivity to be so misinterpreted. First, I discuss a particularly important meta-analytic technique specifically designed to distinguish germane signals from noise and then briefly introduce a much broader group of methods collectively known as Statistical Parametric Mapping.

Meta-Analyses

It is now well appreciated from efforts to meta-analyze a body of experimental results that there is a great deal of variability in the responses. For example, Figure 2.1 shows the near universal distribution of the raw locations of activation peaks produced by a collection of individual experiments that were subsequently pooled in a meta-analysis. Although each of the selected experiments might

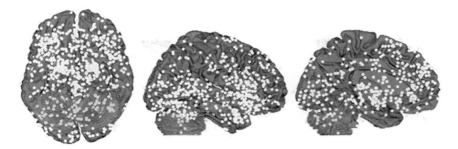

FIGURE 2.1 Activation Peaks After a Meta-Analysis of Emotion

(From Kober, Barrett, Joseph, Bliss-Moreau, Lindquist, and Wager, 2008 with the permission of the publisher)

produce a relatively modest number of activation peaks, as those identified by each experiment are added to the pool, virtually all of the brain is eventually activated by widespread distributions of peaks.

The prevailing current assumption is that hidden within this seemingly random distribution of activation peaks are dense subclusters of especially salient and statistically significant responses that can be identified by appropriate analyses. These significant clusters are presumed to probabilistically represent the brain regions most closely associated with the cognitive task under study. The problem is, thus, a classical, if complex, signal-from-noise extraction protocol that assumes that wherever there is a statistically significant cluster of brain responses from the individual experiments, that is the region or regions of the brain associated with the cognitive task—in this exemplar case, single word reading. The method developed by Turkeltaub, Eden, Jones, and Zeffiro (2002) is currently the most popular method[5] for extracting these subclusters to filter out significant clusters of activation peaks from the insignificant "noise"—the activations that fell below the significance criterion.

This approach ignores an important aspect of the problem—what are the "noise" peaks (i.e., those not significantly grouped into clusters), and what should we do with them? Are they true responses being generated by the variability in the definition of the target cognitive processes or random artifacts of the analyses of such a system? Or are they spurious responses emerging because of some nearly random aspect of the brain response that occasionally throws up a phantom peak? In current fact, we really do not know what we should do with these responses; it is not clear that we should simply drop them because of their relative sparseness. Yet, this is exactly what is done when one uses the Turkeltaub et al. (2002) technique as well as all other similar meta-analyses. Here again, the need for well-designed replications might help to resolve these questions. Unfortunately, at the present time, inconsistency is more evident than replication in the current literature.

Other Data Analysis Methods

Turkeltaub et al.'s (2002) widely used method is not the only one developed over the recent decade to process brain image data. Indeed, developing data gathering, extracting, and accumulation methods for functional brain imaging has become a major activity in the field. The basic reason for this commitment of time and energy, as noted earlier, is the poor signal-to-noise ratios typical of the responses recorded with positron emission tomography (PET) and fMRI systems.

This is not the place for a full discussion of the available methods for processing data. Fortunately, an extensive compendium of such methods has been published by Friston, Ashburner, Kiebel, Nichols, and Penny (2007) under the title *Statistical Parametric Mapping*. This volume considers many problems that pose challenges and difficulties to the formal analysis of brain images. These problems range from the need to compare locales in different brains (registration and normalization) to distinguishing valid signals from background noise. The methods for mapping significant brain responses ranged from classical statistical inference, through general linear models, to Bayesian inference. As powerful and effective as these procedures are, it must be remembered that they are essentially designed to process brain image response information, not to model or explain it.

The Friston et al. book is dedicated to the methodology of signal processing; unfortunately, there is a remarkable paucity of patently cognitive neuroscience examples in it. However useful many of these methods may prove to be in measuring, extracting, and consolidating salient brain activities, there are still many conceptual, logical, and psychological issues that are beyond their intended methodological range. In other words, no matter how efficient these methods for the analysis of brain responses may be, they do not become of direct theoretical concern to *cognitive* neuroscience until compared with cognitive processes. The essential point to keep in mind is that just because we can measure something from the brain does not mean that it has anything to say about the mind-brain problem. It has yet to be established that even the most statistically significant imaging data from the brain is a measure of the psychoneural equivalent of a correlated cognitive process. Of course, this is not an unusual attribute of cognitive neuroscience; the difficulty of making the giant leap from correlated to causal is a major factor in all sciences. Nevertheless, the factors that make it difficult generally are enhanced when we are dealing with the mind-brain problem.

The task now confronting us is to determine the relation, if any, between the products—brain images—of these data-analysis methods and our mental activities. Unfortunately, such theories are rare. In the following sections, I consider some specific examples of studies that have not risen to the level of "theory" but that must be considered at best as "prototheories."

The important conclusion to be drawn from the present discussion is that none of these methods for extracting significant clusters of peaks even begins to be a pregnant prototheory of brain organization. However complex they may appear to be, they are only statistical tools for extracting, displaying, and identifying salient data. Nevertheless, there is a subtle implication that the output of, for example, a meta-analysis experiment is something more than well-massaged data. This happens neither often nor explicitly, but a careful reading of many empirical reports indicates that this logical leap occurs cryptically in our thinking more than it should.

2.4 A Sample Macroneural Prototheory

An example of a potential next step in a neuroreductive approach to theory building is illustrated by the work of Uncapher and Wagner (2009). They were interested in determining the brain locations associated with the cognitive process known as episodic encoding, particularly as it was influenced by attention. Uncapher and Wagner based their work on a solid psychological foundation; the phenomenon of episodic encoding has been and continues to be a well-researched topic in psychology. It has to do with how we learn, store, and retrieve memories about life events (as opposed to implicit or nondeclarative learning such as classical conditioning or skill learning). For many years, since the pioneering work of Scoville and Milner (1957), encoding of this kind of learning had been associated with the medial temporal lobe (MTL), the prefrontal cortex (PFC), and especially with the hippocampus.

However, as is so typical of much of this research, as the science progressed, such a relatively localized model as that proposed by Scoville and Milner has been replaced with a more distributed theory of multiple salient locales. In addition to the PFC and MTL, it has now been reported that the lateral posterior parietal cortex (PPC) is specifically involved in the retrieval of episodic memories. However, different regions of the PPC seem to carry out different functions. For example, the ventral regions of the lateral PPC seem to be associated with retrieval of episodic memories, whereas activity in the dorsal PPC enhances the storage of memories by virtue of its attention directing mode.

From psychological evidence, it was also well established that attention plays a very important role in encoding episodic memories (see, for example, Anderson & Craik, 1974). Given the information from the psychophysical experiments and the suggested dual attention role of the PPC, it was a short step to the assumption that there was an intimate relation between the PPC and the encoding of memories. Thus, Uncapher and Wagner (2009) proposed that "multiple parietal attentional mechanisms modulate episodic encoding" (p. 151); in this case, taking a logical step forward from a mere tabulation of the responsive brain regions to a prototheory.

This example of a reductive cognitive neuroscientific prototheory, as Uncapher and Wagner themselves pointed out, is not a theory despite the fact that the work has multiple theoretical implications. What it and other studies like it added to the simple tabulation of responding brain areas was the concept of interconnection. Although one would have wished they had provided us with a summary chart indicating the various components and the ways in which they were interconnected both functionally and anatomically (the valence of these functional interconnections would also have benefitted from such a "map"), this idea was a major step forward from the simple kind of prototheory that merely listed the responding brain locales. The most important aspect of the Uncapher and Wagner work is that it represents an example of a detailed prototheory of cognitively related brain activity formulated as a network of interconnected brain regions.

However, there are some aspects of this next stage of theory building that constrain and limit the applicability of this general method:

1. The general approach to this kind of theory development is carried out at the macroneural level. Despite the large amount of research that has been carried out at this level, it is not at all clear that this is the proper level at which to seek the neural causes of cognitive processes. As noted several times so far in this book, there is a strong prevailing opinion that the mind and its properties are the result of the activities occurring at a much more microneuronal level of action. The links from cognition, to the brain's localized depletion of oxygen, to fMRI images, for example, are not that direct. Whatever correlations between these brain images and cognition may be interpretable in terms of other indirect or even spurious causes.

2. Some of the functional relationships observed in brain imaging experiments are based upon mathematical fictions. It is not well known, for example, that if one averages a set of range-limited, logarithmic curves, the cumulative curve will typically be a power law (Anderson & Tweney, 1997) and logarithmic functions can be produced by averaging hyperbolic functions (Killeen, 1994). Such artifacts of mathematics (i.e., these cumulative functions) can lead to gross misinterpretations of the responses of groups of subjects; for example, to the traditional power law theory of sensory intensities.

3. Some of the most basic aspects of the functional and anatomical properties of these complex brain systems remain underdetermined. The nomenclature that is used to designate areas of the brain (either verbal specifications such as the "lateral posterior parietal cortex," the Brodmann numbered areas, or the Talairach and Tournoux three-dimensional coordinates) do not precisely identify locations on the brain. Nor are the boundaries between different areas as crisply demarcated as we would like. Indeed, it is likely that functions assigned to well-circumscribed areas actually can be made to either retract from or flow over into several adjacent regions as a result of the arbitrary manipulation of the thresholds for significance.

4. More seriously, it is not yet convincingly established that specific cognitive processes are represented by particular areas of the brain or that particular areas have process-specific functions. The data supporting function-specific localization have recently become suspect.

2.5 Nontheories—"Theories" Without Data: The Neo-Neurosciences

Introduction

The nontheories and prototheories discussed so far are, in general, not intended to be explanatory, and are reductionist only to the extent that particular brain regions are tenuously associated with particular cognitive processes. They are, as expressed in the previous discussions, mainly empirical findings; nevertheless they represent a necessary step that may provide heuristics for more complete theories in the future. However, there is another movement afoot that does make some serious theoretical statements, albeit in a data-poor environment. Indeed, this section considers what are currently by their inventors offered as completely new sciences with very sparse empirical foundations. In the place of starting with data that might provide a footing for the theoretical pyramid, it is as if they started with the apex first. This is not a good way to build either a pyramid or a theory.

In the place of data, attempts to create new neurosciences seem to be based on the basic postulates that (1) the brain creates the mind [true enough] and that (2) we know enough about how it does this to link widely disparate activities such as cellular neurophysiology to complex social systems such as macroeconomics [arguably not true]. This section considers this class of nontheory; a class typified by the relative absence of any robust supporting data and a substantial amount of scientific hubris.

With the simultaneous advent of the brain imaging techniques and communication techniques, a level of scientific hyperbole has emerged concerning the mind-brain relationship that may have been unprecedented in modern popular science history. Despite the many technical and conceptual difficulties in applying brain imaging devices to what are plausibly germane brain and cognitive problems, there has been an empirically unjustified rush to apply some vague implications of this emerging technology to a large number of social and cultural activities. Until recently, there had been little opportunity in any of these areas of human inquiry to relate them to neurophysiology; the traditional social sciences being so conceptually, computationally, and empirically remote from the neurosciences. Unfortunately, when it was attempted, the uncertainties of the brain imaging approach were more often than not compounded by equally intractable difficulties and hindrances to understanding among the social sciences such as economics, philosophy, aesthetics, and so forth.

The main motivation for what seems to be unjustified extrapolation of findings from neurophysiological laboratories to, for example, economics, was, therefore, not compelling empirical evidence, but, instead, a normal human desire to extrapolate from whatever limited knowledge of brain function we may have to the mysteries of molar human behavior. The twin facts that information was being recorded from the brain and that our behavior is controlled by the brain suggested to a number of investigators that cognitive neuroscience had crossed a threshold of understanding that might allow it to inform social science. Although there is no question in cognitive neuroscientific circles that the brain is the "organ of the mind" and that all behavior, thought, mental activity, and cognition (including economic decision making) are the result of the intricate ebb and flow of information among the parts of the brain, it seemed unappreciated that the boundaries between the two domains had not yet been crossed by contemporary cognitive neuroscience. It cannot be reasonably disputed that our research has not yet developed to the point that it could bridge the relatively short gap from neurophysiology to individual cognitive activity. Why, then, should we expect that we will be able to bridge the much longer conceptual gap between neurophysiology and economics? Although there has been considerable progress in linking individual human behavioral decision making and economics (psychology will always be extremely proud of the accomplishments of our Nobelist Daniel Kahneman and his colleague Amos Tversky, 1937–1996), there is a paucity of experimental evidence that even indirectly links current neurophysiology to the complex and often irrational way that economic decisions are made beyond, say, analogies of process and confusions of terminology. The putative explanations that claim to have done so, truly, are additional examples of theories without data.

Figure 2.2 is a sketchy, cartoon-like characterization of the multiple levels of mind-brain interaction and the bridges that must be built between each of them. Modern cognitive neuroscientists are at work striving to explain the relationships among the various levels by developing linking hypotheses. Unfortunately,

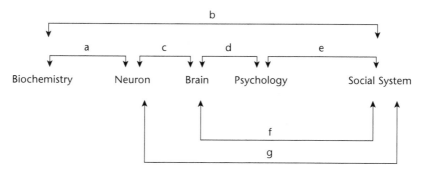

FIGURE 2.2 The Conceptual Links Between Various Levels of Analysis

although a few of these bridges may already exist, others currently appear to be far less achievable than hoped for by proponents of the authors of these neosciences.

For example, as this book testifies, an enormous amount of work has been directed at developing the relation between brain loci activations and cognitive processes in individual human beings. The hypothetical bridge labeled "d" represents possible linking theories between these two levels of analysis. This is the bread and butter of modern brain image-based cognitive neuroscience. It is still debatable, however, just how successful this bridging effort has been, but for the moment, let us accept the empirical fact that we are at least finding some neural *correlates* for cognitive processes between these two levels.

There also has been major progress in bridging the ionic model of neural actions to the electrical responses of neurons—the line labeled "a." Another success is indicated by the line labeled "e"—the relation between individual psychological properties and social systems such as economics as reported by Kahneman and Tversky. This is a relation between two purely behavioral levels and does not include any neuroreductionist postulates, just psychological ones. On the other hand, we still do not have definitive answers to the question of how microneuronal responses are pooled to produce macroneural measures such as the fMRI—the bridge indicated by "c." Such answers may appear in the future but, for the moment, such bridges are just a matter of extrapolation from what are often irrelevant findings.

There are some notable failures from a theoretical point of view that suggest that there are many, if not most, of these bridges indicated in this figure that remain uncrossed despite the fact that there have been some practical successes. As Valenstein (1998) has cogently discussed, the use of psychological active drugs to modify individual behavior is an often successful application based on an almost total absence of explanatory theory. The specific nature of the explanatory bridge (line "b") remains unexplained despite the fact that drugs are often successful in treating mental illness.

Most germane to our present discussion, however, is the fact that robust empirical data linking neuronal activity (line "g") or brain image data (line "f") to such social systems as economics are very hard to find. The main instances of supportive literature for these theories are based more on functional analogies than any definitive empirical linking of the levels. Indeed, without stretching logic too far, it can be argued that there is *no* evidence that macroeconomic behavior is yet reflected in any neuronal or image data findings now available. Experiments that correlate these neural responses with such social concepts as "value" do not satisfy this need because the meaning of the term "value" changes from one analytic level to another; what the word "value" denotes to a single human in terms of survival may be vastly different from what it means to an economist studying the stock market. Nor, for that matter, to my knowledge, have any experiments that alter macroeconomic behavior by metabolic or disruptive techniques involving the manipulation of transmitter chemicals, other drugs, electrical or magnetic stimulation of the brain, short of the massive disruption of normal behavior, ever been carried out.

Although I am sure that a good proportion of the proponents of some of these neotheories might reject this assertion, a close examination of the literature shows that the postulated relevant links between neurophysiology and economics are actually little more than speculations or imaginative extrapolations between unbridged levels of analysis based on functional analogies and the ambiguous nature of the meaning of key words.

> A functional analogy is defined as a similarity in the behavior or trajectory of two systems that is not due to a common mechanism. It is the opposite of a structural homology, in which either same or different behaviors can be attributed to a common mechanism.

The initial erroneous assumption (that we were currently in a position to explain social systems behavior with fMRI systems or any other kind of neurophysiological measure) led surprisingly quickly to the creation of a number of what are generously called "neo-neurosciences," and which ungenerously might be better characterized as "pseudo-neurosciences." The main characteristic of all of these new efforts is that they dote on analogies between neurophysiological results and whatever classic cognitive, social, or even theological problems were of interest. A brief list of some of these neo-neurosciences would at least include the following:

- Neuroeconomics[6]
- Neuroesthetics
- Neuroethics
- Neurolaw
- Neuromarketing
- Neuropolitics
- Neurosociology or Neurosocial psychology
- Neurotheology
- Neuroeducation

The exemplar neoscience—Neuroeconomics—that I use in the following critique to illustrate a "theory without data" is based on the assumption that, whatever hypotheses that may be proposed or any correlations observed are still more in the form of limited and distant analogies and metaphors than of robust empirical evidence linking cognition and society, on the one hand, and cognitive processes and brain activity, on the other.

I reiterate, to make my position in this debate absolutely clear, that there is no robust empirical evidence providing support for the idea that the behavior of a single neuron, a particular transmitter substance, or any part of the brain at either the microneuronal or macroneural level, can explain human altruism, economic choice, religiosity, veracity, or any other social or cultural behavioral activity. Few scientists deny the fact that these social or behavioral activities are the product of brain activity. However, in place of either well-founded explanatory theory or ingenious intuitive leaps, neural responses have been loosely related to behavior at the societal level by what are, at best, analogical links. It seems much more likely that the neural mechanisms underlying our ethical, social, and economic decisions are hidden deeply in incredibly complex neural neuronal interactions and brain states to which we currently have no access.

Why this happens is that in some ontological sense, all such neotheoretical attempts must be correct in principle—all human behavioral and mental activities are ultimately attributable to brain activity! To not accept this most basic premise would erode the most basic foundations of cognitive neuroscience and place us on a slippery slope to dualistic thinking. However, contrary to this ontological assertion is an epistemological question whose answer carries a much less positive message. Does the ontological certainty of mind and brain identity mean that the relationship between these two domains of mind and brain are analyzable and understandable in practice? The answer to this epistemological query is "almost certainly not," both at the moment and quite possibly not in the future.[7]

Another answer to the question of why such links between brain-talk and society-talk are so persistent is that they are in part based on linguistic puns—the indiscriminate use of words that have more than one possible meaning! The idea that the science of cognitive neuroscience née physiological psychology was based on linguistic puns was presciently suggested by Bannister (1968). Referring to one of the "non-logical juxtaposition between physiological and psychological concepts," he asserted:

> The use of terms which are a psychological and physiological *double entendre* and which thereby claim integration based on a pun—e.g., the term 'arousal' which is simultaneously used to refer to the physiological state of the reticular activating system and a generalized psychological disposition.
>
> *(p. 231)*

Misleading identifications, analogies, or metaphors of distantly related concepts are, thus, often drawn between words that sound alike and may even have the same spelling but have very different meanings. Thus, the word "cost" has two entirely different meanings in two different contexts—one at the most macroneural level of the stock market and the other at the most microneuronal level of individual neuronal responses denoting very different concepts.

As an example of how this kind of "punning" can lead to the development of what has many of the superficial appearances, but not the substance, of a new science, I now discuss Neuroeconomics; possibly the most highly developed and widely accepted of the neo-neurosciences scientific approaches.

Neuroeconomics: Theory Without Data

Neuroeconomics, as Glimcher, Camerer, Fehr, and Poldrack (2009) represent it, is dedicated to understanding the biochemical and physiological foundations of the macroeconomic and psychological aspects of a set of factors (reward, value, choice, risk, utility, decision making, preferences, and other variables) that they believe transcends many disparate levels of scientific analysis. Lest there be any misunderstanding that practitioners of Neuroeconomics are simply studying the same sort of thing as are more conventional cognitive neuroscientists (the relation between brain responses and individual cognition), attention is called by McMaster (2011) to an unpublished definition of the field by Camerer in which the most macroneural aspects of social interaction are included within the domain of Neuroeconomics:

> The use of data on brain processes to suggest new underpinnings for economic theories, which explain how much people save, why there are strikes, why the stock market fluctuates, the nature of consumer confidence and its effect on the economy, and so forth. This means that we will eventually be able to replace the simple mathematical ideas that have been used in economics with more neurally-detailed descriptions.
>
> *(Comment by Camerer quoted from*
> *p. 115 in McMaster, 2011)*

Neuroeconomics can be seen, therefore, to be an explicit and premeditated attempt to develop a neuroreductionist theory of macroeconomic behavior. It may consist of many derivative steps from the most microneuronal to the most macroneural, but the ultimate goal is to represent macroeconomic behavior with neural primitives. Any hope of achieving such a grand leap from the neural to the economic, I argue, is limited to vague analogies drawn between various kinds of more or less conventional cognitive neurosciences and economic decision making. I further argue that there is virtually no direct or even reasonably remote indirect empirical evidence at the present time linking macroeconomic activity to neural activity.

The chain of explanatory steps and logic suggested by the practitioners of Neuroeconomics that goes from the single neuron to complex social decision making is a very, very long one. It is studded, in the opinion of some (see later examples of critical comments), with weak conceptual links, logical pitfalls, and conceptual landmines of many kinds. Ideally, at each step it would be desirable to explain (i.e., reduce) observations from one level to another in the terms of lower ones. For a full and complete theory, we would wish to know how single neuron activities affect the neuronal network state, how the neural network states produce molar responses such as EEGs or fMRI images, and so on for all of the steps that take us from the neuron to a brain image to the stock market as illustrated in Figure 2.2. For reasons of both practicality and deep principle, however, I argue that such an overarching theory is not likely to be achieved even in the distant future if the leap from fMRI responses to individual psychological processes such as attention or learning is still a matter of doubt. How much less likely will it be to make the leap from neurophysiology to such subtle thought processes as those involved in choosing to purchase a particular bond or stock? The distant hopes that it would be wonderful if we could bridge all of these successive stages or the intellectual challenge posed by such a formidable task are not enough to support the idea of a Neuroeconomics—data are needed. It would be of earth-shaking importance if support for this neo-neuroscience could be actualized for many conceptual, mathematical, and empirical reasons. Unfortunately, it is extremely unlikely to be fruitful despite the enthusiasm of some of its proponents. This is a highly contentious issue, but various properties of the mind-brain system, not the least of which is combinatorial complexity, suggest that building such a long explanatory bridge from neural networks to macroeconomics is implausible.

Even if we could succeed in terms of metaphors or analogies, what of substance might be added to our understanding of economic decision making merely by adding neural language and concepts to macroeconomics remains unclear. In much of the literature in this field, neurophysiological and behavioral topics are introduced together almost coincidentally, primarily because of common or analogous language rather than by virtue of even the slimmest functional correlations.

A major problem with the entire neuroreductionist approach to economic theory is that much of the enterprise is based on ambiguous definitions just as are the terminologies of psychology. The word "Neuroeconomics" means many different things to practitioners in this field of inquiry.[8] For some people, it is a specific science with specific goals; namely, the "neurologizing" of complex social behavior. For others, it is more theoretical. Glimcher et al. (2009), for example, asserted that "the goal of Neuroeconomics is an algorithmic description of the human mechanisms for choice" (p. 503). Could this be a cryptic reference to a descriptive, essentially nonneuroreductive, but mathematical, theory? If so, Neuroeconomics simply defines itself out of existence and reverts to traditional mathematical modeling.

Glimcher (2009) went on to more particular, but mixed, neural and behavioral statements as "Choice, I propose is accomplished in a network that includes the posterior parietal cortex and a number of movement related areas subsequent to it in the motor control stream" (p. 519). This may or may not be correct, but it is unclear how neurophysiological findings might possibly inform us about macroeconomic behavior. It is, again, an example of a theory without data.

In sum, it can be fairly argued, I believe, that there is no scientific basis for the neurologizing of either economics in the sense of the classical meaning attributed to the giants of theoretical economics of the past including Adam Smith (1723–1790), Vilfredo Pareto (1848–1923), John Maynard Keynes (1883–1946), and others given that only modest progress has been made in the neurophysiological basis of decision making by individuals. The conceptual bonds that tie the disparate levels of analysis together are very tenuous.

There is a considerable amount of internal debate about the status of the Neuroeconomics field even among its strongest supporters. There was, for example, an interesting clash of opinion about the future of Neuroeconomics in the Glimcher et al. (2009) book between two eminent psychologists. One is the Nobel laureate Daniel Kahneman (2009), and the other is the psychologist Charles Gallistel (2009). Kahneman, although pointing out the relative rarity of "well identified psychological and neural measures" (p. 523), was hopeful that the union of the two fields is going to be productive from a futurist point of view. The combination of the two fields, according to Kahneman, "will soon play a large role in shaping the concepts and theories of behavioral research" (p. 525). Kahneman's arguments in support of Neuroeconomics are "the high correlation between well-identified psychological and neural measures" (p. 523), "analogies" (p. 524), and "the findings of Neuroeconomics research have generally confirmed the expectations of behavioral economists" (p. 524). None of these arguments are especially compelling from my point of view. However, Kahneman also acknowledged the conceptual problems of correlation and their "equivocal" nature.

Gallistel, on the other hand, was far less enthusiastic and supportive of any neuroreductionist approach to economic behavior. Although he acknowledged that the field is still at a stage where "contemporary efforts [are trying] to turn . . . aspiration into knowledge," he also pointed out "that the objects of analysis and the terms in which the analyses are conducted at one level (economics) have no obvious referents or definitions at the other level (neuroscience)" (p. 419).

Other scholars have also expressed skeptical comments about the Neuroeconomics enterprise. Bernheim (2009) discussed the potential pitfalls in the steps that have to be taken to establish a robust Neuroeconomics. Gul and Pesendorfer (2008), in an extensive analysis of the concept of Neuroeconomics, made the following criticisms of the new field:

1. The topics studied in Neuroeconomics are not the ones usually studied by traditional economists.
2. The hope that we will be able to distinguish between alternative economic theories may not help traditional economists unless there are neural postulates in such a theory—*which there usually are not.*

3. The likelihood of building an economic theory from the bottom up (i.e., neurophysiologically) is remote.

4. At the present time, ideas are mainly flowing down from the economic and psychological levels to the neurophysiological ones. Neuroscience has not yet provided any ideas or concepts that have flowed upwards to either psychology or economics. As usual, it is the behavioral sciences that inform the neurophysiological ones, and not vice versa.

5. It is notable that although a number of associations have been made between behavior and neurophysiology and between individual behavior and macroeconomics, there are few, if any, such links between neurophysiology and macroeconomics. Nevertheless, these links are supposed to be the distinguishing goals at the core of Neuroeconomics.

6. Many of the ideas are based on animal behavioral studies. The animals are used as "models" of the more complex economic behavior exhibited by humans. Whether this notion of "model systems" works in this case as well as in biological studies of diseases has not yet been established.

7. There is major doubt about the practical application of neural measures to study learning simply because of the cumbersome nature of most of these neurophysiological measuring devices. It is unlikely that we will be able to use a MRI system, a microelectrode recording device, or a microanalytic chemical measure to monitor learning. However, this is mainly a technical issue and new engineering developments often surprise us.

(Summarized from Gul and Pesendorfer, 2008)

Other cogent criticisms of the Neuroeconomics concept can be found in Fox and Poldrack (2009). Despite their general approval of the enterprise, they identify other potential problems. Following a solid and extensive introduction of a mathematical model of prospect theory,[9] the authors mention what they consider relevant neuroscientific evidence. However, in doing so, they raise many problems with the effort to link neuroscience findings with the abstractions of prospect theory. Two of the most germane of the problems they identify are as follows:

1. The difficulty of developing "clean comparisons." That is, the assurance that independent cognitive variables are precisely enough defined. This was also known to them as the problem of "isolating task components." For example, they suggest that "utility" is an ambiguous term that may involve many explicit as well as cryptic influences.

2. The previously mentioned tendency to "infer mental states from neural data in a careless, unqualified manner."

(Summarized from Fox and Poldrack, 2009)

McMaster (2011), to note another example of a critical evaluation of Neuroeconomics, discussed various reasons why he was skeptical of the whole Neuroeconomics movement. These include the following:

1. Divergent interpretations of supposedly comparable experiments
2. Underdetermination of hypotheses by the experimental data
3. The frailty of the subtraction method, which depends on a "linear, unidirectional systemic model of the brain" (p. 121), whereas the brain is a nonlinear system with major feedback, feed forward, and lateral loops.
4. The "mereological" fallacy; that is, imbuing a property only attributable to the whole upon a part.
5. A lack of conceptual linkage between concepts such as emotions and social institutions

(Summarized from McMaster, 2011)

Others who have joined the critical attack on Neuroeconomics include Fumagalli (2010), who reviewed some of its basic concepts. I have already mentioned that he considers the "definitional heterogeneity" of what the field is about as a critical weakness in establishing its bona fides. In addition, van Rooij and Van Orden (2011) examined a number of recent reports in the current literature and noted the wide range of discrepancies between interpretations of what are supposed to be comparable experiments. Their comment is based on the lack of consistent results available so far. It is, thus, fundamentally an empirical critique; the kind that has special weight.

A few daring investigators have gone as far as associating specific neural structures to features of prospect theory. The most specific statement of the neural embodiments of the kind of risky decision making underlying Neuroeconomics has come from Trepel, Fox, and Poldrack (2005). They suggest extremely specific associations between the factors in Kahneman and Tversky's prospect theory and certain brain regions and structures. Their hypothetical associations are summarized in Table 2.1.

Despite the specificity of these associations of risky decision making and neuroanatomy, Trepel, Fox, and Poldrack (2005) were extremely cautious in presenting these associations. In their words:

> There is a large body of suggestive evidence regarding the neural basis of decision-making, and it is possible to at least weakly associate neural systems with the different components of prospect theory. Further work will be needed to better judge the degree to which this theory provides leverage towards understanding of the neural basis of decision making.
>
> *(p. 46)*

This moderate statement with its cautionary terminology (e.g., "suggestive" and "weakly") is itself a compelling critique of Neuroeconomics. These terms highlight

TABLE 2.1 Hypothetical Associations between Neural Structures and Prospect Factors

Component	Prospect theory feature	Brain areas	Neurotransmitter systems
Value function	• Representation of value		
	– Anticipated gains	– Ventral striatum – ACC	• DA (increase)
	– Anticipated losses	– Amygdala	
	– Experienced gains	– Dorsal/ventral striatum – VMPFC	
	– Experienced losses	– ACC – Amygdala – Dorsal striatum	• DA (decrease)
	• Loss Aversion	• Amygdala	• NA
Weighting function	• Diminishing sensitivity – Overweight low *p* – Underweight high *p*	– Ventral striatum (hope?) – Amygdala (fear?)	• DA (hope?)
	• Subcertainty		• 5-HT (impulsivity)
Representation	• Framing	• DLPFC • ACC	
	• Editing	• DLPFC • VLPFC	• DA • 5-HT

(From Trepel, Fox, and Poldrack, 2005, with the permission of the publisher)

Abbreviations: Dopamine (DA), Serotonin (5-HT), Noradrenaline (NA), Dorsolateral prefrontal cortex (DLPFC), Anterior cingulate cortex (ACC), VLPFC (inhibition), Ventromedial prefrontal cortex (VMPFC).

the speculative nature of any neurophysiological interpretation of behavior and the uncertainty that pervades the field. However, Trepel, Fox, and Poldrack's most compelling criticism of these putative associations is the fragility of the empirical links between specific brain structures and the components of this kind of behavior. The associations of brain regions and the components of prospect theory presented here are based on very uncertain extrapolations from a very inconsistent literature. Nevertheless, their work has the advantage of being specific as opposed to some of the remote generalities and metaphorical statements made by others in the field. Whether their model is technically correct in detail is almost inconsequential at this point in the development of cognitive neuroscience. The real issue is, can we establish a more accurate set of associations between specific macroeconomic components and equally specific neural mechanisms? In the opinion of some of us, there is no possibility that an updated, accurate, and empirically robust version of Table 2.1 is likely to emerge in the near or distant future.

In sum, many of the proponents of Neuroeconomics are hard pressed to establish the relevance of any kind of neurophysiology (macroneural or microneuronal) to this proposed neoscience (or, for that matter, any other of the neoneurosciences), in light of the extremely long logical and empirical leaps from neurophysiological findings to the stock market. Indeed, there are relatively few well-established links between what are even adjacent levels of analysis. Until those links are established, it seems unlikely that we will be able to use brain images or neuronal responses to explain such social systems as Macroeconomics in neural terms. In general, therefore, I argue here that there is a paucity (if not a total absence) of robust empirical data capable of developing relations between single neurons, neuronal networks, and brain images, on the one hand, and the activities of macroeconomic systems, on the other. While imagination, heuristics, and extrapolations are important steps in any science, clearly there is a long way to go before robust empirical and conceptual links that go beyond simplistic functional analogies and linguistic puns will be established between macroeconomics and neuroscience.

2.6 Interim Summary

Of one thing, we can be certain: Cognitive neuroscience in general is at a very early stage of development in dealing with the mind-brain problem. As such, there is a relative paucity of robust neuroreductive theoretical explanations of cognitive processes. In place of what may be an unobtainable overarching theory of how the brain (at any analytic level) produces cognitive and other mental activity, a number of approximations I designated as prototheories have emerged. Some of these prototheories may possibly be necessary initial steps towards theories of which we can only imagine at the present time. However, the lacuna that is represented by current theory has led to an explosion of popular hyperbole as well as an outburst of somewhat strained attempts to link the neurophysiological and cognitive domains in a manner that is empirically unsupportable. This does not mean that we should abandon all plausible lines of research, but it does suggest that extra caution is needed in dealing with putative explanations of mind-brain relations.

The idea that either macroneural or microneuronal data can contribute to our understanding of either individual decision making, of macroeconomics, or of any other social science, remains controversial, however widely it may be accepted. The logical leap from the neural to the social levels of discourse is much too long despite the misleading role of a superficially similar terminology. For example, the idea that the factors of macroeconomics might map directly onto neurophysiological functions and processes is almost certainly a gross oversimplification of the complexity of both the nervous system and its role as the psychoneural equivalent of cognitive activity. In general, I argue here that there is a paucity (if not a total absence) of *robust* empirical data capable of developing relations between either macroneural and microneuronal levels of analysis, on the one hand, and social and behavioral functions, on the other. Although imagination, heuristics, and extrapolations are important steps in consolidating the findings of any science, clearly there is a long way to go before compelling empirical and conceptual links transcending simplistic analogies and linguistic puns and representing the neural underpinnings of behavioral processes such as learning, perception, or decision making will be established between cognition and neurosciences. Although there are some preliminary suggestions that transmitter chemistry, single cell, EEG, and magnetic resonance imaging (MRI) techniques might ultimately be useful simply as correlated biomarkers, the field is still in too primitive a state of development to justify the substitution of neurophysiological measures for direct measures of behavioral or mental abilities at the present time. Too much of the current corpus of understanding is incomplete, inconsistent, and replicated. The following quotation from Harrison (2008) seems to me to be especially insightful:

> Understanding more about the how the brain functions *should* [i.e., in principle] help us to understand economic behavior. But some would have us believe that it has done this already, and that insights from neuroscience have already provided insights into economics that we would not otherwise have. Much of this is just academic hype, and to get down to substantive issues we need to identify the fluff for what it is.
>
> *(p. 303)*

This brings us to the end of this chapter. By use of a few key examples, I review here a variety of prototheories that do not, in my estimation, rise to the level of even first approximations to adequate theoretical statements. Neuroeconomics and others of its ilk are frail prototheories because the supporting data do not exist that take us beyond the speculative dreams of their founders. However, the main reason for both the flimsiness of theory and the paucity of evidence in the fields discussed here are conceptual; there still seem to be insurmountable barriers standing between the most robust postulates of neurophysiology and behavior. Vague or metaphorical similarities excite but do not reflect the vast differences in measurements, language, and the degree of development of their respective sciences. There is so much to be learned about the basic postulates of each of these sciences and even more about the bridges relating them to justify the creation of any of these neosciences. Countervailing the intrinsic difficulty of the mind-brain problem, there exist profound, enthusiastic, and completely understandable aspirations to provide reductionist answers to questions about some of the most important properties of human nature.

Before discussing the current status of macrotheory in cognitive neuroscience, it is now useful to clarify the conceptual background by making some of these issues explicit. This is the purpose of Chapter 3.

Notes

1. The most powerful interpretation—literal equivalence—in all of their properties is the manner expressed by "identity" theorists such as Place (1956) and Feigl (1958). In identity theory, cognitive and neural processes have the strongest possible relationship—the one is the other.

2. Other techniques for studying the temporal response properties of the brain (e.g., the EEG) or its constituent neurons (e.g., the microelectrode) are also available, but my main concern here is with brain images. Those alternatives force us to think along other dimensions—temporal patterns in particular.

3. As I develop in Chapter 5, the basic idea that there are significant, localized activation peaks is now under attack. New experiments described there suggest that the "peaks" may be artifacts of sample size and statistical analysis procedures that prejudge the existence of the peaks. In fact, if these studies are correct, peaks of brain activity identified by brain imaging equipment are artifacts in which our statistical techniques have created a false orderliness out of what are actually stochastic processes.

4. The conclusions of these three articles are taken from a more complete list of similar research publications presented in Uttal (2012). My readers should look there for other examples of this kind of barefoot empiricism.

5. The method developed by Turkeltaub et al. (2002) is only one of the several methods now being used to meta-analyze pools of data. Another popular one has been developed by Wager, Phan, Liberzon, and Taylor (2003) and further improved by Wager, Jonides, and Reading (2004).

6. I concentrate my critique here on Neuroeconomics. It is the most highly developed and also exhibits many of the common properties that raise questions about the whole idea of seeking information about high-level social sciences in the responses of the brain. Many of these other neosciences could have been critiqued on similar grounds, but I hope the general point is made by this discussion of Neuroeconomics.

7. It is appropriate at this point to reiterate another very important part of my argument. The inability to link mind and brain at the microneuronal network level (where the origins of mind are most likely to be found) is not because of any fundamental "in principle" barrier, but it is entirely due to a practical one—the basic fact of complexity that the number of neuronal network elements associated with even the simplest cognitive process is very likely to be combinatorially intractable. I repeat, this obstacle is not overcome by the availability of modern supercomputer technology.

8. Definitions of Neuroeconomics vary substantially from author to author. See Fumagalli (2010) for a list of five different meanings of the word. He refers to this as "definitional heterogeneity" (p. 121).

9. Prospect theory, as interpreted in the modern form by Kahneman and Tversky (1979), is a mathematical theory of how people make decisions in uncertain situations involving both gains and losses.

3

CONCEPTUAL ISSUES

3.1 Introduction

In previous chapters, I discuss a number of prototheoretical activities that in my judgment did not satisfy current criteria sufficiently strongly to be designated as true neuroreductionist theories. In this context, I suggest that although an enormous amount of data has been forthcoming, there is relatively little synthesis or integrated theory building underway. Instead, the prototypical question asked in any brain imaging experiment (which is the main empirical basis of modern macrotheories) is, where is a response elicited when we activate a particular cognitive state? Limited to the degree that the empirical data are consistent, most current prototheories are dominated by simplistic metaphors and analogies, computationally intractable speculations, or narrowly circumscribed hypothesis testing that add little real understanding to our knowledge of the mind-brain relationship.

In particular, current cognitive neuroscience theorizing is dominated by macroneural studies of the activity of relatively broad regions of the brain recorded mainly by brain imaging systems. The resulting data typically are used to indicate where in the brain activity is generated by particular cognitive stimuli and tasks. The reason for this macroneural focus is that this is what the brain imaging systems do—they measure *where* in the brain correlates of some cognitive task-related activity may appear, and this is the main tool available to researchers.

The question now arises: Is the flood of current brain image-based cognitive neuroscience findings going to remain a collection of unrelated facts incapable of being synthesized into a coherent and integrated overarching theory of brain organization? Or, on the contrary, is the present situation just the necessary early exploratory stage of a budding science that will eventually join the pantheon of the greatest intellectual developments of human history? In order to answer this rhetorical question, we have to understand the clash between macroneural concepts and prototheories, on the one hand, and conjectures about the microneuronal nature of brain activity, on the other. Where we are now can be summed up in the following two assertions. First, macroneural experiments have provided a plethora of empirical evidence that are interpreted in terms of localization and specialization of function of macroscopic regions of the brain. Second, and alternatively, many cognitive neuroscientists believe that cognition is actually a process emerging from the collective activity or states of a multitude of interacting microneuronal structures, the neurons—the minuscule cells that make up the brain. According to this conjecture, the process should be studied microneuronally, but not in terms of individual neurons, which individually don't have the information capacity to represent the emergent content of a unified experience of some cognitive process. What does have the necessary information capacity is the ensemble of individual states of the network of idiosyncratic neurons—the Hebb conjecture. Unfortunately, the sheer numerousness of components invoked in this mode of analysis precludes experimental manipulations (see the Martin et al., 2000, microneuronal criteria for a "proof").[1] Thus, because of their availability and the possibility that they provide a cumulative sum of the activity of the microneuronal components, we turn to macroneural signals as an experimentally convenient means of representing the essential information. This approach is followed despite the fact that there may be irreversible pooling (and, thus, information loss) of the necessary microneuronal information. In sum, the current consensus is that although the Hebb microneuronal conjecture is probably correct, and although we need "micro" tools to study it, modern technology mainly has given us "macro" tools. In this chapter, my goal is to consider the conceptual issues that lie behind what is now the most popular approach to neuroreductive theory—Macroneural Connectionist Theory (MCT).

A Macroneural Connectionist Theory (MCT) is a statement of the manner in which the action of a system of macroscopic nodes and interconnections (typically developed at the gross level of brain images) represents or encodes cognitive processes.

A Microneuronal Connectionist Theory is a statement of the manner in which the action of a system of microscopic neurons and their interactions represent or encode cognitive processes.

Then, after considering the conceptual issues, I move on to describe how these issues speak to modern MCT theories by describing several alternative types of MCTs.

3.2   Prologue—The Conceptual Issues

It is very important to emphasize that the issues that I deal with here are those that specifically relate to macroneural measures of cognition. However, there are many others that do not specifically involve cognition that are equally important. Physiological and anatomical uncertainties abound in brain science. One of the most interesting is how the macroneural BOLD-based signals reported in an fMRI experiment (or, for that matter, any other mass activity of the brain) arise from the huge number of individual neurons participating in the mental activity. It is presumed that these signals arise from the accumulation or summation of the activities of a host of individual neurons. How this basic physiological accumulation occurs remains uncertain. Deco, Jirsa, Robinson, Breakspear, & Friston, 2008, in a review of this question, have suggested how the microneuronal spiking activity of neurons can combine to produce macroneural patterns of brain activity; a hypothesis also supported by Mukamel et al. (2005).

Others (e.g., Ekstrom, 2010; Logothetis et al., 2001) have suggested that it may be the local potential activity rather than the spike activity that is somehow accumulated to produce the brain's macroneural responses. However, either source, spike or local activity, by virtue of their cumulative nature, throws away nearly all of the microneuronal data that may be critical in understanding cognitive effects.

Surprisingly, it is also possible, according to Ekstrom (2010) that spike, local, and BOLD responses are not as tightly linked as is currently believed. He suggested that his

> models provide guidance in predicting when BOLD can be expected to reflect neural processing and when the underlying relation with BOLD may be more complex than a direct correspondence.
>
> *(p. 233)*

Ekstrom points out that there is an emerging body of evidence that suggest that BOLD signal can be "dissociated" from the underlying neural activity under some conditions. His admonition is well taken; especially when we try to use fMRI signals as a measure of the neural activity accompanying cognitive activity. In his words:

> While fMRI is a potentially extremely useful and valuable tool, caution is necessary in interpreting its results particularly with regard to making direct inferences abut underlying neural activity. More studies need to be conducted, particularly in brain regions outside the visual cortex.[2]
>
> *(p. 241)*

Whatever is the basic mechanism of pooling, it is important to remember that the intended effect of using pooled data is to make that which is intractable, tractable. Neurophysiologically, the idea is that,

> The activity in populations of neurons might be understood by reducing the degrees of freedom from many to few hence resolving an otherwise intractable computation problem.
>
> *(Deco et al., 2008, p. 2)*

Psychologically, the concept is that somehow the combined activity of the many kinds of components of the brain must produce a unified phenomenological experience.

I have organized this chapter's discussion in the context of issues that are germane to the interdisciplinary concerns of cognitive neuroscientists. My attention is directed at attempts to transcend the empirical data and highlight the often overlooked conceptual issues that permeate this field. These questions are less often asked than are those underlying the vast empirical effort. However, conceptual, if not philosophical, issues such as those now presented are at least as important in dealing with the problems of cognitive neuroscience as are the anatomical and physiological ones.

Issue 1

Is the macroneural level at which brain imaging devices provide data the proper arena for carrying out the quest for a theory of mind-brain relationships? If not *the* proper level, is it at least a plausible approach with which to pursue a theory of mind-brain relationships? In other words, are the fMRI responses evoked by cognitive stimuli related closely enough to associated cognitive activity to offer some promise of even a partial explanation of how brain functions are transformed into experiential ones?

Issue 2

Is the information about neural activity in the form of the BOLD signals produced by brain imaging devices adequate to serve as the foundation of a meaningful theory? The problem is that these macroneural responses are inseparable accumulations of the responses of a myriad of idiosyncratic individual neurons. As a result, much of what many think is salient and necessary information about brain activity is lost during the imaging process. Is what remains germane to the development of putative theories, or is it just the meaningless residue of otherwise irretrievably lost data? In particular, are what many cognitive neuroscientists believe to be the salient microneuronal information processes recoverable from these pooled responses? The relation between the microneuronal and the macroneural connectionist levels of analysis remains uncertain, as we saw earlier. At the very least, almost all of what is thought by Hebbian-type theorists to be the critical microneuronal information is lost, first by the physiological, and then by subsequent statistical pooling of data. We must ask, therefore: Is there any way to go between the macroneural and the microneuronal in either direction? In more familiar terms, will either the "top-down" or "bottom-up" strategy lead to a mind-brain theory?

Issue 3

Are the data being obtained by brain imaging devices consistent and reliable enough to be trusted as evidence for cognitive theory building?

Issue 4

Are the identified brain regions, locales, activation site, modules, or "nodes" in which activations are supposed to be selectively evoked valid indicators of the macroneural organization of the brain? Do they represent, as postulated, function-specific, specialized, localized, and segregatable regions of brain activity? Alternatively, to the contrary, are they merely stochastically fluctuating peaks of a broadly distributed field of activation in which nearly every brain region participates in every mental activity? In other words, what is the current status of the local-distributed debate? In short, do localized nodes of activation adequately characterize the organization of the cognitive activated brain? To put it most baldly: Do nodes exist?

Issue 5

Are the bands of white matter interconnecting the putative functional regions, nodes, or locales of the brain so general that they interconnect all regions with all other regions? Or, to the contrary, are these bands selective and specific enough that the properties of their specific trajectories can be considered to be a part of the theoretical process? In other words, do selective interconnection patterns exist, or is every region interconnected to every other region?

Issue 6

Is there sufficient support for the more or less arbitrary segregation of cognitive processes into what psychologists have conventionally called "functional modules" or "faculties" that could possibly map in any direct way onto localized regions of the brain? If not, it will become extremely difficult to associate the vaguely defined areas of the brain with the equally vaguely defined cognitive processes.

Issue 7

Are the potential theories truly driven by the empirical data and not just by whatever is the prevailing metaphor, Zeitgeist or, even worse, whatever technology is currently available? The issue in this case is that definitive empirical evidence of mind-brain relationships has been unavailable for so long, and the desire to provide such a theory so persistent, that a plethora of marginally supportable prototheories has emerged. These prejudgments can presumably allow our view of ambiguous data to be so unconstrained that it is possible, if not likely, to construct a completely erroneous theory from what are essentially insignificant responses. In short, are our prototheories driven by data or by preexisting biases?

Issue 8

Are available brain responses sufficiently robust that we can distinguish between the two main currently contending theories—localization and distribution—of mind-brain relationships? At present, many investigators still adhere to the classic "phrenological" theory of localized, function-specific regions on the brain. A variation of this premise is that the brain is made up of systems of strongly interconnected macroneural "nodes" that collectively encode or represent cognitive processes. Others argue that brain mechanisms are broadly distributed and functionally nonspecific. A persistent problem is that it is still not clear if the two ideas are distinguishable by the available data.

Issue 9

Is it possible to "analyze" the macroneural brain with existing mathematical tools? One estimate (Modha & Singh, 2010) holds that the 383 regions of the macaque brain are interconnected by 6,602 long-distance connections. As I suggest throughout this book, simple combinatorial calculations suggest that this complex problem is intractable at the microlevel of individual neurons. Thus, there are likely to be problems of tractability, computability, combinatorics, and complexity that may preclude analysis at any level of the human brain. This should not be surprising; some comparable problems in other sciences are well known to be intractable and thus beyond theoretical realization or practical implementation. Is it likely that any mind-brain theory of data may encounter as intractable a challenge to analysis and interpretation as those already encountered and accepted in the physical sciences?

Issue 10

The relation between psychological and neurophysiological theories is still the core of cognitive neuroscience. But two basic conceptual questions are not yet resolved. The first is, can psychological responses inform neurophysiology? The second is, can neural responses inform psychology? As pervasive as is the assumption that both of these questions can be answered in the affirmative, a deeper examination suggests that there remain unanswered conceptual challenges to both of them. Negative answers, needless to say, would be extremely significant in defining the nature of a future cognitive neuroscience.

There are, of course, many other conceptual issues beyond these 10. For example, a related methodological issue concerns the nature of theories—should they be probabilistic or deterministic? Are both possible? Are neither? Similarly, the dynamic and adaptive properties of the brain may also bear on the problem of theory building. If the brain is constantly changing as it adapts to new experiences, are our experimental techniques adequate to keep up with both the magnitude and the temporal dynamics of brain activity?

These 10 issues (and many others of less immediacy) stand in the way of the development of a plausible mind-brain theory. To begin to understand these conceptual difficulties, we have to start with an introduction to MCT, the most popular current way of melding macroneural brain imaging data and cognitive activity into a plausible theory.

3.3 Introduction to MCT

Given the issues identified in the preceding section, it is obvious that developing an explanatory theory of correspondences between cognitive processes and brain image–type data is going to be not only a challenging empirical task, but also a major conceptual challenge. Nevertheless, there are some obvious harbingers of just what a macroneural theory may look like, at least in the immediate future. The technical properties of the brain imaging technique, for example, dictate that any such theory is necessarily going to be mainly limited to some version of an answer to the "where" question. That is, whatever theory emerges based on brain imaging technologies is going to have to be framed in terms of the spatial organization of the brain. Beyond this generalization, whether spatial data at this macroneural level of analysis are going to be an adequate entrée to a deep understanding of mind-brain relationships cannot be determined at present. It is possible, as I noted previously, that the brain imaging technique operates at a level of neurophysiological response pooling that will always obscure what we will learn to be the critical microneuronal information. The persistent possibility, given our current state of knowledge about brain organization, is that the idea of localized, function-specific nodes of activity is an illusion produced more by the vagaries of technique than the reality of the biology of the brain. These are important issues simply because the ultimate theoretical context is not likely to be one based on macroneural measurements, despite all of the past work that has been done in this busy field. Full and overarching theoretical explanations are more likely to be eventually framed in the properties of microneuronal networks that are currently obscured by their very complexity and the limits on our technological capabilities.

Be that as it may, it is what I designate as the MCT that dominates current mind-brain theory and, therefore, it is this approach that appropriately demands our first attention. It is the purpose of this section to describe the manner in which MCT have evolved in the past 30 years since the fMRI systems became available. The kind of emerging theories described here is, as it is in most sciences, a natural product of the techniques available to us. It is not yet a neuroreductive theory of how the mind emerges from brain activity nor is it a priori a plausible theory of how we can use neurophysiological data to manipulate behavior or "read the mind." It is, at best, a description of regional brain locations and their interactions and, for the moment at least, of correlations between macroneural responses and cognitive activity. The rock-bottom goal in developing an MCT is to determine how particular macroneural patterns of macroscopic interactions might be related to cognitive processes; however, we are a long way from achieving this goal.

For an MCT (i.e., one based on the interaction of macroneural nodes) actually to be implemented, it requires positive responses to all of the issues described at the outset of this chapter. A negative answer to any of the 10 issues listed should raise serious questions about this kind of cognitive neuroscience prototheory at the outset. If too many are negative, MCTs would be reduced to nothing more than descriptions of the data and other kinds of armchair speculation—an approach that is antithetical to the ideology of current cognitive neuroscience.

Given, for the sake of argument, robust affirmative responses to all 10 of these issues, what would a putative MCT look like? There are several obvious answers to this question. First, it would have many of the characteristics of an increasingly common model of brain activities—a distributed network of many interacting macroneural parts (nodes in the language of graph theory) interconnected by a system of tracts (edges also from the same graph theory context). Models of this kind of macroneural theory of brain organization have traditionally been offered by a number of investigators over the years. Perhaps the best known, as well as one of the earliest, of the MCTs is the one proposed for emotional responses by Papez (1937) shown in Figure 3.1. This iconic MCT model is characterized by anatomically localized regions of the brain and their known interconnections, especially the notion of feedback from one region onto itself by what may be very indirect routes. A centrally important property of the Papez circuit is that there are both cerebral and brain stem regions involved. It is, therefore, a model that incorporates broad regions of the brain. Indeed, newer work suggests that many other regions[3] of the brain are involved in its emotional role, including additional cortical and subcortical regions that were not part of Papez's original theory. It is also important to remember that inclusion in the Papez circuit does not preclude a particular center from performing other functions—a property that is characteristic of most current MCT-type theories.

Many other MCTs have been proposed over the years by Van Essen, Anderson, and Felleman (1992) for vision; Kaas (2004) for audition; Jones, Fontanni, and Katz (2006) for gustation; Squire (1992) for memory consolidation; Thompson

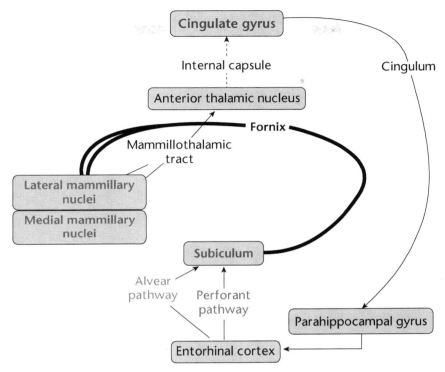

FIGURE 3.1 A Classical Macroneural Network Theory: Papez's (1937) Original MCT Theory of Emotion

(From Wikipedia article on Papez circuit, used with the permission of their Creative Commons License Grant.)

(2005) for cerebellar learning; and Ashby, Ennis, and Spiering (2007) for perceptual classification.

All of these MCTs have certain common properties. First, most obviously, they all consist of multiple activation regions, or nodes. That is, there is a near-universal appreciation among investigators these days that there are no isolatable anatomical regions responsible for a single separable cognitive process.

Second, the nodes are interconnected by a complex network of tracts. Often these networks have been well demonstrated anatomically and are presumed to link the nodes into a unified system.

Third, the nodes are multifunctional. They are not limited to their participation in a particular process but may have different functions in different networks as required by the cognitive task at hand.

Fourth, the interconnecting tracts are typically assumed to be bidirectional and widespread throughout the brain.

The implication of this type of theory of macroneural network organization is that the brain mechanisms of even very simple cognitive processes are not localized but are widely distributed throughout the brain. Large portions, if not the whole brain, are presumably involved in any mental activity according to the precepts of the MCT approach to brain organization. However well such models have served us, we are reminded by Kaas (2004) that, like all of other such network models, they are speculative structures based on data of varying quality and completeness. Indeed, Papez's theory was largely based on an intuitive leap from his anatomical observations to the cognitive (emotional) concept it represented.

A common characteristic of MCT theories, past and present, as we have seen, is that they are composed of what are intended to be anatomically and functionally demarcated nodes. It is important to point out, however, that these nodes are very different in concept than the classic "phrenological" assignment of complex psychological processes (e.g., acquisitiveness) to unique brain and demarcated regions that was popular during the first phase of brain imaging research. Most modern theories today accept that the regions of the brain depicted in their diagrams are involved in many different cognitive processes. By assuming that the cognitive processes they instantiate are produced by the activity of multiple interconnected regions and that these regions may have other functions in other MCT-type systems, all traces of phrenological-like function-specificity should have been eliminated from our thinking. Any attribution to specific cognitive functions solely to specific regions of the brain would be incorrect according to recent thinking about brain organization.

Another common implication of all of these connectionist-type theories (and the anatomical data) is that they are selectively interconnected. That is, not all parts of the brain are connected to all other parts. This eliminates any possibility of a traditional equipotential mode of brain action. To the degree that the nodes are actually functionally circumscribed regions of the brain (and not just the peaks of a more or less continuous distribution raised to prominence by relatively high probabilistic thresholds), the brain cannot be considered to be functionally or structurally homogeneous; there is a degree of anatomical as well as functional specialization of various degrees assumed in all of these prototheories.

A further common feature of MCT is that there is two-way communication either directly or indirectly from one node to another. Even if neurons are physiologically constrained by the monodirectionality of neural conduction, it is usually assumed that there is some kind of feedback between nodes *if, in fact, nodes actually exist.* Direct two-way interaction is not necessary: Indirect connections may be implemented by means of secondary circuits that loop through other nodes back to the point at which the activity of the system is initiated. It is likely that potential pathways for internodal interaction are far more complex than suggested by any available MCT theory. A single line on a graphic representation of a theory may actually represent diffuse bands of interconnecting tracts that pass from their origins to their destinations and then back again in multiple steps through both direct and indirect pathways. The point being that the best network models currently being developed at the macroneural levels are certainly oversimplifications of the actual nature of brain organization.

Depending on the particular MCT theory with which we are dealing, there may be multiple nodes at each level of information processing as well as multiple parallel paths between nodes. Because of this kind of organization, brain systems of this type always are subject to some kind of feedback from the outputs to the inputs; in other words, centrifugal activity from the higher levels of the nervous system to lower levels. This feedback offers serious challenges to any effort to determine the hierarchical[4] structure of the system. However, it also illustrates another common conceptual feature of all of these network theories— they are all essentially parallel processors and thus any analysis of their operation will be very difficult to obtain.

It is also important to reiterate and make explicit another universal aspect of MCT theories—the level of analysis at which they are constructed. Based mainly as they are on macroneural findings (ranging from lesioning to fMRI data), they can speak only to phenomena, structures, and processes at that macroneural level. Few expect that the MRI-based techniques will be able to provide information at the microneuronal level at which the idea of a "network" means something quite different—a network of neurons is quite different from a network of macroneural nodes. Even the most optimistic technology prophets do not assume that fMRI systems will be able to operate at the micro-anatomical level for large numbers of individual neurons.[5] Thus, at the present time, the MCT approach does not incorporate theorizing about the properties of synapses, axons, and dendrites and their interconnections except as indirect measures or to emphasize the neural nature of the theory.

The basic concept of current MCT theories, therefore, involves large-scale nodes approximating the size of Brodmann areas and connecting tracts involving vast numbers of individual axons. The responses of individual participating neurons and synapses are hidden in the cumulative fMRI measures as information is pooled, averaged, combined, and integrated. Even if the technological tour de force of improving the fine functional resolution of brain imaging devices to the microneuronal level could be accomplished, we would then face the computational problem of dealing with the very large numbers of neurons and their synaptic interconnections that must be involved in cognitively relevant neuronal networks.

In sum, the kind of macroneural data obtained with fMRI systems are, in the large, useful only to particular kinds of explanatory models and theories, those classified here as MCTs. A further complication is that it is also likely that the network of macroneural brain regions involved in a cognitive process may be dynamic—a moving target—changing from moment to moment. Like the excellent adaptive system that it is, the brain is constantly adjusting not only its processing strategies but, almost certainly, also selecting, from moment to moment, the most appropriate neural mechanisms required to solve a problem or select a response. From this point of view, there is no certainty that the same cognitive task will be responded to with the same network from one day to the next; there are many ways to carry out a task, and it seems all too plausible that the slightest stimulus change or past experience difference could drastically affect which neural mechanisms were being recruited. Indeed, it seems likely that no static, unchanging theory of cognitive processing could ever be tenable except as a first approximation. At the very least, we know that experience alters the state of the brain. Thus, there may be no single MCT-type "theory" that works for more than a moment. The few studies (e.g., Aguirre, Zarahn, & D'Esposito, 1998; McGonigle et al., 2000; and Miller et al., 2002) of intrasubject reliability that have been carried out reflect the transitory nature of brain responses even at the intrasubject level.

3.4 Appraisal-Responses to the Conceptual Issues

Within the context of the discussion just presented, we can now begin to at least tentatively examine the 10 conceptual issues posed earlier in this chapter. Some of the issues can currently be rejected or confirmed on empirical grounds; others await empirical support and still others depend on logical disagreements and arguments that will probably always be contentious. The purpose of the forthcoming discussion is to express the current view of the answers to the mix of issues that confront cognitive neuroscientists in their search for an explanation of the mind-brain problem.

Response to Issue 1—Is the macroneural level the correct one to analyze cognition?
There is a persistent empirical question concerning how direct the relation is between the macroneural responses measured with brain imaging technology and cognition. Should data eventually converge on consistent answers to questions about which parts of the brain are active in which cognitive processes, some kind of a more or less "direct" relation might be assumed to exist. Exactly what is the nature of that kind of "relation" depends on concepts and ideas that probably do not currently exist. Possible meanings of the word may include "literal identity," "correlation," "concomitancy," and "complementary," as well as "no observable functional relation." At worst, macroneural responses may be more a function of the anatomy or physiology of the brain rather than the cognitive processes generated by stimuli. In this case, the brain would be responding to inputs in much the same way that a cymbal responds in a particular way to a physical stimulus—there is a response, but it is determined only by the impulse of the stimulus (the fact that an event occurred) and the physical properties (as opposed to the informational properties) of the brain. In such a situation, the brain's response may not signify anything about the information content of the stimulus

or the resulting cognitive process. Instead, brain imaging signals would have to be considered to be artifacts, third-order correlates, or biomarkers rather than being causally related to cognition. If this view is correct, then the macroscopic level at which data of this kind are produced may be entirely inappropriate and irrelevant to the decoding of the brain's representation of cognitive processes.

Response to Issue 2—Are macroneural data sufficient to determine cognitive processes?
It is not yet known whether what many cognitive neuroscientists believe to be the essential microneuronal, neuronal net information underlying cognition is preserved in macroneural signals. If the Hebbian (Hebb, 1949) idea of neuronal states, cell assemblies, and phase sequences modulated by synaptic efficacy changes is generally correct, than cognition can be found or understood only at the microneuronal level of the individual states of neurons in the neuronal network. If this is the case, combination, mixing, amalgamating, or pooling (alternate names for the common property of all macroneural measures to integrate, pool, summate, or average lower level responses) may destroy the critical microneuronal information we need to decode the brain's role in creating mind. If this is true, then any technique in which the respective brain activation maps produced by control and experimental conditions are subtracted from each other—a strategy ubiquitous throughout the literature—would lead to ambiguous conclusions.

This widely overlooked fact arises simply because two brain images may be identical at the macroneural level despite the fact that the underlying microneuronal network states may be completely different. This is an inevitable result of combining or pooling data—the fine details of any responses are lost as some kind of an average or integrated value is generated. The fundamental problem in the present context is that investigators cannot go back to extract the micro-details of neuronal network activity from the macroneural measures. It would require a recovery of information that for all practical purposes no longer exists. This is fundamental; to assume otherwise would be a violation of the second law of thermodynamics. A fundamental premise of cognitive neuroscience must be that none of its theories violate physical principle and laws. If this point of view is correct, then it is not possible for macroneural responses to serve as a foundation of a cognitive neuroscience theory.

Response to Issue 3—Do macroneural data replicate?
Because of the great variability of current research findings, there remains considerable doubt about the reliability of brain imaging data. Not only is there a question about the data, but also the validity of the entire statistical hypothesis testing approach used in evaluating cognitive and neuroscientific findings has been repeatedly challenged in past decades. (Recent challenges have come from Bakan, 1966; Bakker & Wicherts, 2011; Ioannidis, 2005; Lambdin, 2012; Nieuwenhuis, Forstmann, & Wagenmakers, 2011; and Simmons, Nelson, & Simonsohn, 2011.) Although relatively rarely explored, the few explicitly comparative studies of reliability and consistency that have been carried out

report a great deal of intrasubject, intersubject, interexperiment, and meta-analytical variance. (See my extended discussion of this matter in Uttal, 2013, and a brief discussion of this topic in Chapter 5 of this book.) It is also the case that, in general, it is becoming increasingly obvious that the criterion p values used for statistical significance testing in psychological and neuroscience research are probably much too lenient and should be made considerably more rigorous. (See, for example, Simmons et al., 2011.) Finally, Carp (2012b) has recently suggested that the inadequate way in which brain image methodology is reported in the contemporary literature obstructs attempts to compare experiments to evaluate their reliability.

Response to Issue 4—Do nodes exist?
Emerging observations are clearly relevant to the question of whether the nodes in MCT-type theories actually exist as real anatomical or as functional entities or are just convenient fictions. For example, the shape and size of the "nodes" or statistically significant clusters of activation areas that are purported to be regions of activation do not correspond to the nomenclature of any of the traditional region-defining systems (e.g., the Brodmann, 1909, nomenclature or the verbal specification of anatomical regions by such phrases as "inferotemporal"). Instead, the nodes or brain regions of interest constitute a new functionally defined macroneural "pseudoanatomy" that does not necessarily correspond to anatomical, chemical, or architectonic systems used to define functional regions of the brain. Furthermore, even in a perfectly random distribution of activation peaks, there are likely to be some clusters of activation peaks that will appear to be significant "nodes" should one incorrectly choose too modest a criterion for significance.

Statistical significance is a very peculiar measure; incorrectly selecting the arbitrary criterion level drastically affects both false positive and correct rejection scores in a complementary fashion—the more "hits," the more "false alarms." In such a case, the pattern of activation on or within the brain might actually be unrelated to cognitive stimuli[6] yet by chance produce the appearance of activation peaks, that is, nodes. Furthermore, as many others (e.g., Andreski, 1972; Bakan, 1966; Killeen, 2005; Lambdin, 2012; Meehl, 1978) have repeatedly pointed out (unfortunately, without much effect on current thinking in the field) statistical significance is not tantamount to theoretical significance or even to empirical validity.

An important aspect of the problem of identifying and defining nodes, there-fore, is that, from a network point of view, what constitutes a node is arbitrary. Sporns (2011), for example, distinguishes between four types of nodes (random, random modular, hierarchical modular, and hierarchical modular-map), any one of which can represent the same data. Which one best represents the data depends on statistical estimates of the mean and standard deviations as well as arbitrary decisions about modularity.

The point is that what constitutes a node can vary considerably depending on the judgment or proclivities of the investigator. Depending on arbitrary criteria, there may be one, few, or many nodes in a putative MCT. Finally, the very existence of discrete nodes is challenged by the recent work of Gonzalez-Castillo et al. (2012) and Thyreau et al. (2012); topics to be extensively discussed in Chapter 5.

Response to Issue 5—Is the brain universally interconnected by tracts or are the connections specialized and selective?

Despite the arbitrariness and fragility of the concept of a node, we now have unequivocal evidence of the high level of anatomical interconnectedness of the various regions and centers of the brain. Modha and Singh (2010) summarized an enormous amount of data describing the interconnections among the various regions of the brain of the macaque monkey.[7] Their summaries were based on the results of 410 tract-tracing experiments and involved 383 brain regions and 6,602 connections. For our purposes, the point being made by their work is that the brain is not uniformly interconnected. Instead, there are regions of high and low interconnectivity suggesting some kind of underlying order. Nevertheless, the indication is that there is some kind of regular organization at the anatomic level more detailed than every place being connected to every other place. One of the tasks that lie ahead is to establish what the nature of these specific interconnections may be.

Of relevant interest is that Modha and Singh also conclude from their work that the prefrontal cortex, although often reported to be activated by cognitive activity, does not seem to have a particularly high density of interconnections. Modha and Singh described a somewhat smaller and more tightly integrated network that seems to be more specifically involved in cognitive processes. All in all, their work strongly supports the anatomic postulate of a widely, but not universally, distributed pattern of interconnecting tracts.

Response to Issue 6—Can cognitive processes be parsed into functional modules?

Among the most difficult problems for any MCT of cognition actually has little to do with the neuroscience side of the equation. Instead, a perpetual and daunting problem for researchers interested in neural-cognitive comparisons lies on the cognitive side. Specifically, our psychological constructs are not precisely enough defined so that we can look for what are purported to be their neural correlates with strong enough assurance to claim that certain cognitive modules actually encode or instantiate meaningful parameters of mental activities. Indeed, the imprecision of definition of cognitive states may be the weakest link in the chain of experiments and logical steps that lead from cognition to MCT theories. The problem is that psychological terminology is deficient in specificity, not only in its denotation of its constructs but also in ability to distinguish between constructs. Thus, any experiment designed to explore a process such as emotion would find it difficult to do so independently of the perceptual, attentive, and response aspects, all of which are parts of the emotional process. Furthermore, such relationships are not even stable. Slight differences in experimental design may invoke major differences in both cognitive phenomena and brain image responses. Furthermore, our inability to define our terminology leads to difficulty in reporting in the published literature exactly what were our methods and variables (Carp, 2012a) so that surprising results can be verified.

Furthermore, how experimental subjects cognitively evaluate the assigned task may change the results even though the experimenter may have thought that the independent variables—the stimuli—were adequately constrained. Our control over covert cognitive states is nowhere as precise as those used to study sensory or motor processes.

Response to Issue 7—Are theories driven by data or by the Zeitgeist?
Another major source of confounding in cognitive neuroscience research (and all other scientific studies) is that all levels of experimental design and, therefore, to a significant degree, all of the results obtained are driven by previous work, ideas, and theories. The truism "that we stand on the shoulders of giants" is certainly valid. Science moves ahead on a foundation of earlier work, which not only guides empirical findings but also sets the current intellectual milieu. Indeed, conservative adherence to earlier work is considered to be an important aspect of science providing stability and resistance to premature paradigm change.

However, there is also a negative side to this historical progression of data and ideas—the previous theoretical perspectives provided by the "giants" can blind us to the significance of new accomplishments and, thus, perpetuate obsolescent points of view. Tradition and history can establish a compelling and influential Zeitgeist, or consensus, view that may be very powerful in determining what and how we go about our research. Kuhn (1962), for example, pointed out the great difficulties in changing the "paradigm" of a science. The consensus that is popular at the moment is extraordinarily influential. Changes occur only when contradictory information becomes so overwhelming that it cannot be denied without injecting logical chaos into current theories. Some paradigms (e.g., localization), especially those in cognitive neuroscience, seem to live on far beyond the time that contradictory evidence demands a change in perspective.

The influence of the current Zeitgeist and "iconic" experiments is abetted by the complexity of the systems, the arbitrariness in decision criteria, and the simple human conservative refusal to appreciate change when it is thrust upon them in the constant wrestling with the natural world to discover its secrets. What we do today is also influenced by the open-endedness of many cognitive neuroscience theories, which allow a great deal of internal inconsistency and all-too-easy adjustment by simply adding degrees of freedom to our theories to accommodate contradictory findings.

Response to Issue 8—Can we distinguish between theories?

Although many of my colleagues would not agree with the point, it is entirely possible that the entire idea of localized, narrowly circumscribed nodes[8] may be a remnant of the postulates of centuries-old phrenology, a field long discredited by standard science.[9] In a field of such complexity and variability as cognitive neuroscience, prejudgments of what is expected can misdirect our attention, exert potent influences on current thinking, and, ultimately, produce spurious results. Indeed, the number of potential biases in a field such as cognitive neurosciences is considerable. I shall not belabor the obvious here but only note that in my earlier book (Uttal, 2012) I devoted two full pages to a partial listing of the multiple sources of bias that currently permeate cognitive neuroscience experiments. Many of these biases were the outcome of strongly held beliefs or existing paradigms on the part of cognitive neuroscientists. With respect, I should point out that the currently accepted research approach (e.g., the use of the fMRI as a way of localizing cognitive function in the brain) is accepted by many, if not most, investigators in this field with little questioning of its fundamental assumptions. Little attention is paid to evaluation of its reliability, analysis of its fundamental postulates, or empirical-based criticisms of this pervasive research strategy. In the poor signal-to-noise ratio environment of modern cognitive neuroscience, it remains uncertain how much of our data is objective and how much is based on prejudgments imposed upon us by those "giants" of the past and their persisting influences on the present.

Evidence is now accumulating that suggests that the brain is responding over broadly distributed areas even when no reportable cognitive activity is going on. This has been referred to as "default" activity by Raichle et al., 2001 and by Raichle and Snyder (2007) or "resting-state" activity by Wang, Zuo, and He (2010). Default responses involve a number of brain areas that decrease their activity when a person is actively thinking or being stimulated by a stimulus.[10] The regions typically associated with this default activity are the posterior cingulate cortex and the ventral anterior cingulate cortex. According to Greicius, Krasnow, Reiss, and Menon (2003), these brain areas are interconnected into a subnetwork of their own. The background, or default activity, of the brain is not always considered when the responses to experimental and control conditions are compared. Most important is the fact that additional noise is introduced by the rest, or default, activity that greatly diminishes our ability to determine what is correlated signal and what is noise.

Another special problem arising from the presence of default activity is that many of the neural responses attributed to stimuli may result not from the specific effect of the cognitive state being studied but from the general effect of any stimulus as the brain shifts between resting and active states. Furthermore, because default activity may also vary with the cognitive state, the role of a control condition in any experiment may be conflated with what may have to be considered intrinsic instability.

The net result of these considerations and others discussed elsewhere in this book is that the data we are using to distinguish between local and distributed may be inadequate to distinguish between these alternative patterns of organization. There is sufficient arbitrariness and such a wide and arbitrary range of organizing this data that arriving at a robust and unique solution to the local-distributed issue may not be possible.

Response to Issue 9—Is the brain too complex ever to be analyzed?
The complexity of the brain's responses is such that powerful mathematical tools will be necessary to make sense of what borders on chaotic or stochastic responses or to detect faint signals in noise. Indeed, the basic assumption underlying MCT-type theories is that by some appropriate analysis we will be able to understand the function of a system of interconnected nodes. However, it is not at all sure that this will be the outcome. Mathematicians such as Hilgetag, O'Neill, and Young (1996) have raised questions about the utility of methods to determine the ordering or hierarchy of complex networks of nodes and connections. They pointed out that there are theoretically 10^{37} possible arrangements of the 32 visual areas of the brain identified by Van Essen et al.(1992). Proposed hierarchical orderings were evaluated on the basis of the number of anatomical constraints (i.e., the observed connections) the model violated. Applying computer analysis techniques to develop the ordering produced no unique hierarchical solution (i.e., a unique model accounting for all of the data). Furthermore, simply providing additional anatomic information led to an ever larger number of possible models. Hilgetag et al. (1996) concluded,

> Thus, the physical hierarchy is indeterminate, No single hierarchy can represent satisfactorily the number and variety of hierarchical orderings that are implied by the anatomical constraints.
>
> *(p. 777)*

Although not claiming that the situation is fundamentally indeterminate, Ramsey et al. (2010) also emphasized the enormous number of configurations that a simple directed graph (typical of those formulated in the form of an MCT) can be higher than 2 billion for as few as 10 nodes. The exact numbers depend on the nature of the interconnections, but, clearly, distinguishing one true macroneural connectionist theory from the hoard of alternatives is not an easy task and, given the numbers, may be impossible. The intractability of the combinatorial problems involved in mind-brain studies remains an open issue. However, there are suggestions that some of the questions being asked by cognitive neuroscientists have already been demonstrated to be unanswerable. It behooves us to consider what is already known in other fields. (See Karp, 1986, for a discussion of the effects of complexity and randomness on the computability and tractability of even relativity simple systems.)

Response to Issue 10—Can psychological theory inform neural theory and vice versa?

One of the most important conceptual issues of all is the relationship between neurophysiological and psychological findings. The issue has been formulated in two related questions. First, can psychological findings inform neurophysiological concepts and, second, its inverse twin, can neurophysiological data inform psychological theories? The answer to this first question is that psychological theory makes cognitive neuroscience possible. Without the guidance of psychology, there could be no cognitive neuroscience; neurophysiologists would have nothing specific (i.e., an observable behavioral response, at best, or a verbal report, at least) for which to search. Thus, the answer to the first question is clear and hardly controversial—psychology informs neurophysiology.

On the other hand, there is a considerable debate whether neurophysiology can inform psychological research. The issue can also be dichotomized. Given that no one has yet provided a robust example[11] of fMRI data actually resolving a psychological issue or informing a "pure" psychological theory, the question arises—is this a practical problem because the science is still young, or does it reflect an "in principle" barrier between neurophysiology and psychology?

One active participant in this debate is Coltheart (2006, 2010) who has argued that, although we cannot predict the future, there is yet no evidence that suggests that any fMRI data have directly or indirectly provided any support for any particular theory of a cognitive process. Mole and Klein (2010) also have contributed to this argument concerning the role that brain images may play in informing psychology. Their main point is that demonstrating consistency is not the same thing as proving a theory or a hypothesis.

Others have joined in the debate concerning how much fMRI data can inform psychological processes. I discussed this issue in an earlier book (Uttal, 2013), highlighting the debate between an opponent (Coltheart, 2006) and a proponent (Henson, 2006), and need not repeat those views here. Others who feel strongly that brain imaging data can inform psychology are Aue, Lavelle, and Cacioppo (2009). The issue has also been raised in a special issue of *Perspectives on Psychological Science* introduced by Mather, Cacioppo, and Kanwisher (2013a). In a separate article (Mather, Cacioppo, and Kanwisher, 2013b, these three investigators have suggested that there are at least four ways in which fMRI findings can inform psychology:

1. Which (if any) functions can be localized to specific brain regions?
2. Can markers of Mental Process X be found during Task Y?
3. How distinct are the representations of different stimuli or tasks?
4. Do two Tasks X and Y engage common or distinct processing mechanisms?

(pp. 108–109)

All of these would be legitimate answers to the challenge made to the ability of fMRI findings to inform psychology if it were not for the fact that all are really alternate versions of the basic "where" question assuming some kind of localization of function. Some investigators now agree that simple localization of cognitive process in function-specific portions of the brain cannot provide the foundation of a neuroreductionist theory of cognitive processes. One reason is that discrete localization is less and less frequently observed. Another is that even if there were robust evidence of localized function, it would not speak to the problem of how these neurophysiological mechanisms were implemented to produce cognitive activity. Thus, the controversy continues. It is a sign of some progress that this issue is now being debated; a few years ago, it would not have been considered to be worthy of comment.

Whatever future contributions neurophysiological findings may or may not make to cognitive understanding, it should be clear that nothing could happen unless the cognitive theories have specific neurophysiological components (Coltheart, 2013). Because most attempts to model cognition are descriptive and nonreductive, it seems that neurophysiology "informing" psychology is still more of a hope than an accomplishment.

Finally, there is the central problem permeating this entire discussion of determining the cognitive function of a brain node. However successful we may be in determining the nature of the structural and functional interconnections among what may be correlated activation areas in the brain, this does not serve the goal of unraveling the complexities of the neural mechanisms encoding psychological functions. Indeed, it seems that great progress may be made in the study of the anatomy of brain networks using powerful tools of network analysis without contributing to the problem of how cognition is represented by these neural networks.

In an instructive tutorial on brain networks, Bullmore and Sporns (2009) introduced the basic ideas of complex brain networks. They showed how MRI, fMRI, EEG, and MEG methods can elucidate both the structural and functional organization of the brain. They also listed a number of network measures that can help to describe the organization of networks, but it should be remembered that a list of network properties does not constitute a theory, but is, at best, a primitive prototheory. Their work, unfortunately, is almost totally devoid of any cognitive correlates beyond mention of Alzheimer's and schizophrenic diseases. Even then, they note that there are "inconsistencies between existing studies" (p. 194). In summing up their article, Bullmore and Sporns conclude the following:

> A related question concerns how the parameters of complex brain networks relate to cognitive and behavioral functions. One can make an intuitively reasonable claim that high clustering favors locally specialized processing whereas short path length favors globally distributed processing; but the empirical evidence is almost non-existent.
>
> *(p. 196)*

Obviously, great progress in neuroanatomy and neurophysiological function can be and has been made concerning the physical properties of the brain without contributing anything to the mind-brain problem, which is the core theme of cognitive neuroscience. Indeed, as I noted earlier, there is no a priori reason that we should expect that the modules of cognition defined by the protocols of experimental psychology should map directly onto modules of the brain; Bullmore and Sporns's work testifies to this point. Their strong implicit admonition is that one should raise questions about alternative hypotheses before designating any brain area or node as a repository of any particular cognitive function.

Hanson and Halchenko (2008) specifically made this point when they criticized the assignment of the cognitive process "face identification" to the anatomical "fusiform face area" (a region of the brain at the ventral intersection of the boundary between the occipital and parietal lobes). They argue that this area is not "uniquely diagnostic for faces" (p. 486) but can be reused in a variety of different functions. This idea of multifunctionality as a general property of any brain region is gaining wide acceptance in cognitive neuroscience circles. It adds further complexity to the development of any theory that seeks to associate specific cognitive functions with specific brain regions.

3.5   Types of MCT Theories

With this conceptual analysis in hand, we can now consider what variations there might be in the formulation of MCT theories. Three types can be identified:

1.   Localized Functions
2.   Distribution With Function-Specific Nodes
3.   Distribution Without Function-Specific Nodes

Localized Functions

Although it has so far proven to be difficult even to find a reliable biomarker of such subtle cognitive dysfunctions as autism, cognitive neuroscience researchers continued to seek tighter relationships between brain responses and mental activity. One might well ask, if we cannot find reliable biomarkers, what chance is there of unearthing signals that actually reflect causal relationships? Nevertheless, the search goes on and has been particularized in the last few decades in the debate between localized and distributed theories. The localized theory proposes that the neurophysiological responses to a cognitive task are constrained to narrowly circumscribed cerebral regions. This theory suggests that each part of the brain has some specialized and possibly independent function-specific role. On the other hand, the distributed theory proposes that the brain responses associated with particular cognitive processes are spread over broad swaths of the brain. Considering the current status of the evidence, it seems clear that the answer to this question must now be phrased in the terms of broad distribution. Although many current investigators report unique, localized representations, this probably is due to statistical manipulations (such as the use of too high a threshold) rather than to the realities of the response.

The traditional theoretical approach to the relationship of macroscopic brain regional activations and cognitive processes dates back to the phrenology of Gall and Spurzheim (1808). No one nowadays gives credence to their "bumps on the skull" theory, but the basic underlying assumption of what was at their time a very popular enterprise—that there are narrowly circumscribed regions on the brain (as reflected in the bumps on the skull) specialized to carry out specific cognitive processes—still motivates, albeit implicitly, many cognitive neuroscientists. The idea of distinct localized regions, each with a distinct cognitive function, persisted until the last decade's eruption of brain imaging studies that showed that brain activity was much more broadly distributed than would support any kind of an extreme localization theory.

The basic "phrenological" idea of localized brain regions representing specialized cognitive processes characterized the entire cognitive neuroscience enterprise for years prior to the development of PET and MRI systems. This history cannot be overlooked in any historical view of the science. Its influence can be seen in the older techniques of experimental brain surgery as well as in the emphasis put on localized trauma cases. Experimental brain surgery and trauma cases both played the same game—determine what cognitive or behavioral dysfunctions occurred when a part of the brain was removed by intent or by accident. The prevailing theory was that when an association was found between a damaged region and a cognitive activity, that region was ipso facto the locus of the missing cognitive function.

Simplistic high-level cognitive neophrenology of this kind was abated by what clearly were observations of localized brain function in the sensory and motor domains. The discovery of the occipital visual area (Munk, 1881), the mapping of the somatosensory homunculus (Woolsey, 1952) and the auditory areas (Tunturi, 1952) as well as what seemed to be dedicated speech areas (Broca, 1861; Wernicke, 1874) were uncritically extrapolated to models assuming similar localized brain mechanisms for higher level cognitive processes such as thinking, rage, or affection. However, as I have repeatedly pointed out, these sensory and motor input-output mechanisms differed in major ways from cognitive processes. Typically, they were elicited by well-defined physical stimuli, required simple discriminative judgments, and were probably better considered as transmission rather than representational systems. Therefore, we should probably consider them to be poor models of the much more complicated higher level cognitive processes.

It was with the rush of new data from the brain imaging devices that these simplistic models of function-specific and localized brain representation of cognitive modules began to fall apart. The typical pattern of PET and fMRI responses to cognitive tasks turned out not to be a single or a few demarcated places on the brain, but rather a multiplicity of poorly defined regions. Furthermore, no region was function-specific; all had multiple functions. The basic empirical fact emerging from this kind of research was not a version of neophrenological localization, but, rather, of a wide distribution of multiple activations.

Lindquist, Wager, Kober, Bliss-Moreau, and Barrett (2012), among others, also came to the conclusion that there is no basis for any kind of function-specific localization. They summarize their results concerning emotion with the following statement:

> Overall, we found little evidence that discrete emotion categories can be consistently and specifically localized to distinct brain regions. Instead, we found evidence that is consistent with a psychological constructionist approach to the mind: a set of interacting brain regions commonly involved in basic psychological operations of both an emotional and non-emotional nature are active during emotional experience and perception across a range of discrete emotional categories.
>
> *(p. 121)*

What this pattern of activations should have implied is that regardless of the cognitive process being considered, many, if not most, brain regions—not a single one or a few—are activated. It now seems beyond reasonable contention that the brain's response during a high-level cognitive process is made up of a distributed system of many different multifunctional locales or regions. The extent and the nature of this distribution are not yet definitively known for any cognitive process, but there is little doubt that the evidence for distribution heavily outweighs that for localization. This does not beg the question of what these responses mean in terms of the representation of cognitive process; it only adds further support to the argument that the old hypothesis of narrowly localized, function-specific nodes can no longer be considered to have any validity. The amount of additional evidence to support this conclusion is now overwhelming. Distribution, not localization, must be the foundation of any future theory of mind-brain relationships.[12]

At this point, we consider two alternative theoretical directions that theory can take from this seemingly irrefutable empirical result. One, the system of nodes approach, preserves something of the neophrenological tradition by maintaining that although the brain response to any stimulus or task is broadly distributed, it can still be characterized as a system of discrete and localized nodes, perhaps corresponding to anatomical structures, each of which has a specialized function. The other, the "soft" distribution approach, considers the brain to be more of a boundary-free, undivided system without any function-specific localized regions other than in sensory or motor regions processing. As we see, the evidence to distinguish between these two kinds of distribution is not as compelling as that distinguishing between function-specific localized nodes and a distributed system without them. Indeed, the difference between a system of discrete nodes and a softly distributed system may also depend on an arbitrary judgment. The data are equivocal on this issue, and the difference may be made not so much on the basis of the empirical data, but, rather, on the theoretical orientation of the cognitive neuroscientist. The next two sections seek to clarify the distinctions between these two alternative views of brain organization.

Distribution With Function-Specific Nodes

The idea that different parts of the brain may perform different functions but must cooperate to encode or represent cognitive process is not a new one. One premier example of this approach can be found in the previously mentioned work of Papez (1937) as shown in Figure 3.1.

Papez was an anatomist who had been influenced by previous work in which a resolution of the James-Lange and Cannon-Bard controversy concerning the nature of emotions was sought.[13] Much of the earlier work (prior to Papez's contribution) on possible neural mechanisms of emotions had been directed at the hypothalamus—an example of the tendency to localize this kind of cognitive function within a single portion of the brain's anatomy. Papez, however, as an anatomist, understood that the hypothalamus was heavily interconnected with other portions of the brain. Based on his understanding of the anatomical inter-connections, he concluded that the hypothalamus did not operate alone but rather that "Taken as a whole, [an] ensemble of structures is proposed as repre-senting theoretically the anatomic basis of the emotions" (Papez, 1937, p. 725). In Papez's original system, the "ensemble of structures" included the following brain structures:

- The Hypothalamus
- The Cingulate Gyrus
- The Anterior Thalamic Nucleus
- The Mammillary Bodies
- The Hippocampus
- The Subiculum
- The Parahippocampal Gyrus
- The Entorhinal Cortex

Subsequent research has made it clear that the frontal cortex and other regions of the brain also play major roles in this system. The essential point of Papez's theory was that the salient brain components of emotion were represented by a broadly distributed system of nodes. Indeed, as we have learned more and more about the brain responses, it was hard to find regions that are not involved in emotion.

Similar brain systems have been proposed for other cognitive activities. Thompson (2005), for example, proposed a conceptually similar system for declarative learning and memory that incorporates the follow brain structures:

- Cerebral Cortex
- Hippocampus
- Cerebellum
- Striatum
- Amygdala

Johnson (1995) carries out the same task for visual attention. He lists[14] the following brain regions as involved in this cognitive process:

- Visual Areas V1, V2, V3, V4
- Frontal Eye Fields
- Dorsolateral Prefrontal Cortex
- Basal Ganglia
- Substantia Nigra
- Lateral Geniculate
- Medial Temporal Cortex
- Inferotemporal Cortex
- Superior Colliculus
- Brain Stem

The key idea in this type of theory is that, although a part of a distributed system, the constituent nodes are localized and function–specific to a particular cognitive process. In the words of Posner, Petersen, Fox, and Raichle (1988):

> The hypothesis is that elementary operations forming the basis of cognitive analyses of human tasks are strictly localized. Many such local operations are involved in any cognitive task. A set of distributed brain areas must be orchestrated in the performance of even simple cognitive tasks. The task itself is not performed by any single area of the brain, but the operations that underlie the performance are strictly localized.
>
> *(p. 1627)*

Posner and Rothbart (2007) have renewed this assertion:

> Results of neuroimaging research also provide an answer to the old question of whether thought processes are localized. Although the network that

carries out cognitive tasks is distributed, the mental operations that constitute the elements of the task are localized.

(p. 18)

The idea expressed here of localized and function-specific nodes encoding or representing mental operations still prevails in the context of many distributed theoretical systems. To a large degree, such theories perpetuate the idea that cognition is represented by specialized and localized mechanisms, although each is a component of a distributed system.

The main point made by all of these function-specific, distributed system models is that no single region of the brain is solely responsible for any cognitive process or subprocess. Instead, each of these theories of cognitive-brain relationships incorporates the idea of a system of distributed nodes that heavily interact with each other. Identifying these specific functions of these nodes is a major goal of much brain imaging research these days. Unfortunately, as we see in Chapter 3, the empirical evidence does not support this kind of specificity nor, for that matter, does it support the idea of isolatable functional nodes of any kind.

Nevertheless, investigators continue to attempt to attach specific functions to nodes by various experimental techniques; however, this effort sets a goal that may be contradicted by the data. These networks are all heavily interconnected with multiple feedback channels. As a result, it is rarely possible to determine where an activity is initiated or whether a part of the system is carrying out either a necessary or a sufficient function (Hilgetag et al., 1996). Ideally, it would be necessary to hold the activities of all except one node constant and manipulate its inputs to determine its role in the system. However, for many technical and conceptual reasons this is not possible. The most significant of these obstacles to carrying out the ideal experiment is that it is probable, if not very likely, that it is the activity of the entire system, indivisible into subunits, that actually instantiates the cognitive process. Nor is it possible to excise one component from such a system and attempt to observe if it serves any singular function. For such a strategy to work, it would require a degree of independence of the various nodes from each other in the manner referred to as "pure insertion" by Sternberg (1969) and Friston et al. (1996). Pure insertion implies that removal of a part of the system would leave all other parts functioning as they did originally. This is a highly unlikely possibility; without pure insertion, any research using surgery or the standard subtraction methods used in brain imaging in an attempt to isolate the function of the excised region would inevitably lead to inconsistent and unreliable results. Any effort, therefore, to divide the system into functional nodes, either surgically or psychologically, would be difficult if not fruitless.

The empirical evidence presented in this book speaks strongly against this concept of function-specific nodes in the brain. By far, the predominant finding is that many brain regions are involved in any cognitive processes; thus, they must serve general rather than specific functions. Nevertheless, our persisting opinions concerning the gross anatomical subdivisions of the brain and of localization still lead many investigators to seek to assign specific functions to these nodes or, in many cases, to parts of them.

The persistent idea that the nodes of a distributed system have specific functions can be distinguished from another kind of distributed theory—one that does not carry the neophrenological localization baggage of the past. This alternative theory is discussed in the next section.

Distribution Without Function-Specific Nodes

The function-specific theory discussed in the previous section implicitly makes a strong theoretical statement—localized activity in a group of function-specific locations in the brain is the psychoneural equivalent of cognition. However, the alternative now being considered is that the "strict" localization and specificity of function may no longer be good models of how the brain works. The empirical facts that different cognitive processes can activate different brain regions and that different brain regions may have different functions in different contexts countervails the idea of function-specificity by localized operators.

This brings us to a theoretical approach that eschews both functional specificity and spatial localization. It accepts that distribution is a fact but has a different outlook on what the distributed brain mechanisms are like and what role they play in representing cognitive functions.[15] In an earlier book, I pointed out the following empirical arguments that support a macroscopic theory of brain organization that is neither function-specific nor localized.

Distribution: The review carried out in this present book strengthens the argument that brain image responses to even the simplest stimuli evoke widely distributed responses throughout the brain. Indeed, the prototypical result of most current research is an extensive listing or depiction of many brain regions that are activated by whatever cognitive process is under investigation rather than a few locales. The more data that are pooled, from subjects and then from experiments, the more broadly distributed are the cumulative responses shown to be. In this context, classical function-specific localization is no longer a viable theory simply because localization is empirically denied at the most preliminary level of data analysis. Furthermore, there are several other properties of current research findings that strongly support this alternative of distributed activity without function-specificity. These include the following:

Anatomical Interconnectedness: Anatomical studies of the brain now make it clear that the various regions of the brain are heavily interconnected. It is, therefore, increasingly likely that no brain region could operate in isolation. Diffusion tensor imaging of the brain highlights the multiple bands of white matter that connect even the most distant regions of the brain. Isolated (i.e., localized) responses are, therefore, logically implausible.

Multifunctionality: Scattered throughout this present book is abundant evidence that every brain region responds in many different cognitive processes; none has any unique role in any particular cognitive process. They, thus, must play multiple roles (i.e., be multifunctional) and cannot be function-specific.

Weakly Bounded Nodes: Regions of the brain are neither anatomically nor physiologically precisely demarcated. None of the usual brain anatomy mapping methods (e.g., the Brodmann areas) correspond exactly to the activation regions reported by investigators. Indeed, what constitutes the extent of an activation is arbitrary depending in large part on the thresholds set by the investigator, either with the imaging devices themselves or the statistical methods used to analyze the complex data sets coming from a brain imaging device.

This is not to assert that the brain is completely homogenous in the sense of "mass action" or "equipotentiality" (Lashley, 1950), but rather to acknowledge that the extent of many of the brain regions that might have been considered to be "nodes" are imprecisely, if at all, defined. Thus, the concept of a "node" itself may be a hypothetical construct without hard meaning in this discussion. What we may be talking about is a softly bounded region of the brain in which the boundaries are indistinct and overlapping and the functions general. What appears to be a node to some may be a broad region of the brain to others.

Methodological Sensitivity: Any hope of finding separable nodes with specific functions depends on consistency across methods. If different methods of analysis produce different boundaries, any putative nodes as well as the boundaries themselves, would be of questionable reality. The increasing divergence of the shape and extent of activation regions as one increases the size of the pool of data, a finding typical of meta-analyses, suggests that many brain regions, particularly the regions of the cerebral cortex, may have no unique cognitive functional meaning.

Functional Recovery: The remarkable ability of the brain to recover function after trauma or surgery is another argument against both innate functional specialization and localization. For the purposes of this present discussion, the most important aspect of this ability is that it means that there is no genetic, predetermined necessity for a particular place in the brain to have a particular function. If in need of repair, other portions than the injured one can often take over some functions. Why, then, is it not plausible to consider that whatever associations there are between a particular place on the brain and a particular cognitive function are also not fixed? There is the ever-present alternative of a kind of ad-lib selective adaptation and adjustment over the life span. If so, then a large amount of individual difference between people would be expected— exactly the finding we encountered in this chapter.

Finally, I sum up this alternative version of a distributed system theory of the relationships between the mind and the brain by noting that current evidence supports the following conclusions:

- The brain operates on the basis of a distributed system—many regions (i.e., nodes) are involved in any cognitive task.
- Each node in such a system has multiple functions that can adapt as needed to satisfy cognitive tasks.
- Distributed nodes of a complex are not fixed in terms of their function. They are general-purpose entities that dynamically adjust to the needs of the system.
- Nor are their spatial extents fixed. The regions overlap and have no clear or permanent boundaries, which may change from situation to situation.
- Indeed, the nodes may not exist in any kind of divisible or separable anatomical sense. They may just be softly bounded regions of maximum activity in an otherwise continuous distribution of activity. We may have to consider them as general-purpose computation-capable regions that may be recruited as necessary to represent some cognitive process rather than as function-specific nodes.
- The distributed macroscopic measures obtained with brain imaging devices are almost certainly not the psychoneural equivalents of mind; they are more likely to be cumulative measures of the activity of the vast underlying neuronal networks. These macroscopic measures may actually obscure rather than illuminate the salient neuronal processes.
- It is possible that the distributed responses are not directly associable with cognition. They may preserve some residual information about the neuronal net information processing; however, they do not preserve the critical information and thus, in principle, cannot explain how brain activity is transmuted into mental activity.
- Brain image responses can vary from subject to subject, from time to time, and from task to task. Therefore, they may not represent a sufficiently stable database from which generalities can be drawn.
- The response of any particular region in a cognitive process is to contribute whatever general-purpose information processing functions are needed to execute a process.
- Regions of strictly predetermined function and precise localization are limited to the transmission pathways of the sensory and motor pathways.
- The idea that poorly defined cognitive modules—the cognitive constructs of psychology—map directly onto function-specific, narrowly localized nodes of the brain is not supported by current research.
- Furthermore, the idea that these poorly defined cognitive modules map in any simple way onto the anatomy of the brain is an implicit, but unsupported, postulate of modern cognitive neuroscience. Considering our empirical results so far, there is no a priori reason that they should.
- In sum, brain imaging defined regions of interest may not be related to cognition in the manner that is implicitly assumed by many current cognitive neuroscientists.

3.6 Interim Summary

This discussion provides a conceptual (as opposed to an empirical) context in which we can examine some of the MCT-type theories that have been proposed to explain how the brain might encode cognitive processes. Before discussing several cognitive neuroscience theories of interconnected nodes, in particular, it is important to point out that not all such theories directly pertain to the cognitive aspects of this science. There has been a considerable amount of very successful work germane only to the anatomic and physiological aspects of the problem that does not involve how brain and cognitive processes are related. This is clearly illustrated by the work of Hilgetag et al. (1996). Their analysis and those of others who have dealt with the same problem (e.g., Aflalo & Graziano, 2011; Reid, Krumnack, Wanke, & Kotter, 2009)[16] were concerned only with the anatomic organization of the brain and not with its cognitive properties. This does not mean that these findings may not be useful in some future cognitively related theory. However, the fact that these works are "brain" studies does not guarantee that both are germane to the problem of the neural basis of cognition. It is possible that a purely anatomical theory of brain organization and function could emerge that had no relevance to the cognitive processes being carried on by the brain. Because we are precluded from any neuron-by-neuron analysis by the sheer numerousness and complexity of the neuronal network that more probably lay at the roots of cognition, this may be the best we can do for the moment.

In the main, the understanding of the macroneural properties of the nervous system represents the cutting edge of cognitive neuroscience theoretical developments. It is at this level of analysis that the dominant instruments provide the most data and for which the prototheories are most prevalent. Before I turn to a discussion of particular examples of this kind of preliminary theorizing, I summarize the previous discussion by noting several emerging principles and caveats that must guide anyone whose goal is to develop an MCT—a macroneural connectionist theory.

1. There is ample empirical evidence that the brain is made up of a vast network of microscopic neurons. These neurons are discrete entities, each of which is separated from its neighbors. Communications between neurons are mediated by synapses, molecular structures that allow information to be communicated without intracellular protoplasmic continuity. This general statement, known as the "Neuron Theory," was first proposed by Wilhelm Waldeyer (1836–1921) and established beyond doubt by the cellular staining studies of Cajal (1900). The neuron doctrine also established the necessary nature of the neuronal network and of interconnections at the microneuronal synaptic level. It has been formalized into a specific theory of mind-brain interaction by Hebb (1949). Hebb's

theory, however, only marginally communicates with the macroneural prototheories that are based on brain imaging findings. His hypothetical macroneuronal cell assemblies and phase sequences do not map directly on specific brain structures.

2. At the macroneural level, the brain is also a complex network of much larger but many fewer interconnected "nodes." There is ample evidence that there are multiple interconnecting tracts connecting these regions. These interconnections are not universal but connect specific regions in a specialized and well-defined manner. The brain is not a random engine at either the microneuronal or the macroneural levels—organisms with brains adapt and function very well. Its complexity is so enormous, however, that it appears to be stochastic; that is, at least partially random. The discouraging harbinger is that we may forever be unable to find order in this form of near-randomness.

3. Macroneural nodes may, like the microneuronal ones, also be considered to be parts of a heavily interconnected network. However, unlike the undeniable anatomic definitiveness of the neuron, their size and extent, as well as the functional and anatomical reality of the "nodes," are open to question. These hypothetical nodes are of different sizes, and their boundaries are poorly demarcated. Indeed, what a node is at this level is arbitrary and variable as is their function that may vary from moment to moment.

4. Although it seems undeniably true that in some fundamental ontological sense, cognitive processes (i.e., the mind) must be a function of neural mechanisms, there is no a priori necessity that the psychologically proposed modules of cognition should map directly onto the neural nodes of the brain. How the brain makes the mind remains one of the most important questions of human history as well as one on which much less progress has been made than is generally appreciated. This assertion is made despite the enormous amount of knowledge we have of human thought and brain anatomy and physiology in their separate domains.

5. Much more so than theories in the physical and other biological sciences, all current psychological and cognitive neuroscience theories are fragile expedients cobbled together more by imaginative speculation than by robust and reliable evidence. It is still moot whether the problem of relating neurophysiological evidence to psychological explanation is solvable or intractable.

6. At the present time, although we know a great deal about the anatomy and physiology of the brain and a great deal about cognitive processes, there is a vast gulf between the two domains. There is nothing that portends an overarching solution to the mind-brain problem despite a substantial amount of what is reputed to be relevant research in the field.

7. And, finally, the basic postulate of all of cognitive neuroscience is that, whatever they are, cognitive processes are manifestations of neural mechanisms of the brain.

With this introduction to the conceptual foundations of current mind-brain theory in hand, we can now turn to consideration of current MCT theories themselves.

Notes

1. New developments in computation neuroscience may mitigate this statement to a certain degree. However, no one has yet met the Martin, Grimwood, and Morris (2000) criteria for the establishment of a microneuronal theory of cognition. In a future book, I will examine progress in this field.
2. This allusion to "brain regions outside the visual cortex" is especially meaningful in the context of arguments I made previously. The mechanisms of sensory coding and its corollary—topological representation—are different than the neural processes underlying complex cognitive processes. A substantial part of the reported successes in cognitive neuroscience is associated with visual encoding.
3. I have brought the Papez model up to date in my earlier work (Uttal, 2011).
4. By hierarchical, I am referring to the order in which the parts of such a system are arranged or activated so that which part is causal to the action of another can be determined.
5. Progress has been made in increasing the resolution of specialized MRI systems to the levels of neurons and even to that of molecules. However, these methods for narrowly localized structure do not yet provide the kind of distributed functional information associated with mental activity that cognitive neuroscientists are pursuing. No one expects that fMRI systems can be used to determine which individual neurons are separately contributing to a BOLD signal. At some point, as resolution increases, macroneural responses will become microneuronal responses with their own attendant difficulties obstructing analysis.
6. I exclude from this comment the sensory and motor pathways and regions for which the spatial organization (e.g., topological consistency) is clear.
7. Although these data are for the macaque monkey, Modha and Singh (2010) point out that it is widely accepted that the homologies between monkey and humans are substantial. They and others such as Orban et al. (2006) base their research on the assumption that there are no fundamental differences between the interconnections of the brains of the two species.
8. Indeed, as we see in Chapter 5, neurophysiological evidence for the existence of localized nodes is currently under attack.
9. To be fair, phrenology is considered by some students of the mind-brain problem to have made a major contribution to modern cognitive neuroscience—the idea of localized, function-specific brain regions. This idea, still prevalent in today's thinking, has to be contrasted with the idea of the broad distribution of nonspecific functional areas.
10. Reduction of brain activity when one is thinking or opening the eyes is reminiscent of alpha blockade, one of the earliest observations made by Berger (1929) when he first recorded the human EEG.

11. I am sure that many of my colleagues would disagree with this assertion. However, if one excludes the more peripheral portions of the brain (i.e., the sensory and motor systems) and theories that are essentially descriptive curve-fitting endeavors, this may not be as outrageous as originally claimed.

12. An interesting idea suggested by my colleague John Reich, a social psychologist at Arizona State University, is that very wide distribution of cognitively salient neural activity is supported by the fact that people have only a limited ability to time-share their thoughts. The suggestion is that most, if not all, of our brain resources are involved in any single cognitive process and that it takes that large proportion of our brain's neuronal network to carry out the information processing necessary to instantiate a thought. Thus, because most of the brain is committed to a single thought under this hypothesis, there is not enough extra processing power to think about more than a few things at one time. Of course, this is not the only speculative reason underlying our single-mindedness, but it is an interesting idea.

13. The James-Lange theory argued that emotions were caused by our perceptions of the physiological responses to emotional stimuli. The Cannon-Bard theory argued that our emotions caused the physiological responses.

14. Johnson attributes this model to Rick Gilmore without further citation.

15. My first presentation of this "theory" was in Uttal (2011). In that discussion, I did not use the word theory because it seemed to me that our models were not specific or substantiated well enough to dignify that accolade. I referred to it as a new "metaphor"—a new way of looking at the mind-brain relationship at the macroscopic level. In this book, I have reverted to the use of the word "theory" for consistency with the other topics in this chapter. However, I still believe that current brain models are not so much theories as metaphors that help us to think about the brain. None of them really answers anything about the mind-brain relationship and the question, what is the cognitive function of a given brain area? may be a bad one. Indeed, it is a "point of view" that may be nothing more than a statement of the inconsistency of the whole corpus of brain imaging studies. The degree of unreliability of the findings in this kind of research suggests that whatever correlations may be observed may be artifacts of our methods rather than neural representations of our thoughts.

16. Recent studies on the problem pioneered by Hilgetag and his colleagues (1996) were able to make some progress on modeling the hierarchal organization of the brain networks but only by applying some strong regularization constraints to simplify the problem. This is, of course, a suitable strategy for solving any complex problem, at least approximately. However it does remind us of the enormous complexity of the brain and that intractability lurks around the corner for many of the computational neuroscience ideas that are introduced to deal with complex systems.

4

MACRONEURAL CONNECTIONIST THEORIES OF COGNITION

4.1 Introduction

Despite the consensual agreement that microneuronal networks must instantiate the ultimate psychoneural equivalents of mental activity, there remains considerable effort to study the relation of macroneural responses produced by fMRI techniques to cognitive processes. However, there is considerable uncertainty about how these macroneural responses relate to these magnificent and as yet imponderable mental functions. Clearly, the increasing dominant concept guiding current theory building at this level is that of a "network" of nodes and interconnecting tracts. Nevertheless, despite the enormous amount of data accruing at the macroneural level, the basic fact is that we still have not definitively linked any cognitive process *directly* to the action of any kind of a neural network, macroneural or microneuronal, beyond the bald statement that such and such regions sometimes seem to be activated during certain cognitive processes or that certain neurons seem to behave in concert with certain cognitive processes. As discussed in the previous chapter, there is still no consensus concerning such fundamental issues as whether macroneural responses can have any theoretical implications.

Nevertheless, everything we now know shouts out that networks of neural components at some level or levels must be the underlying neurophysiological foundation of cognition. Unfortunately, a critical review of the current status of the field suggests that because of the complexity of the brain and the vague manner in which cognitive processes are defined, little progress has been made toward an overarching theory of mind-brain relationships. What we have instead are some narrowly defined speculations and a few loose metaphors based on ambiguous and inconsistent empirical findings. Some of these speculations are ingenious and a few may point the way to the future, but none of them carries the weight or promise of a satisfactory solution to the mind-brain problem or even provides the foundations of a good prototheory.

A caveat concerns the use of the word "network." Some investigators use this word in the anatomic manner typified by Sporns (2011). In this context, a network is defined in terms of macroneural anatomical regions and their interconnections, tangible properties that can be measured or estimated. Others use it in a much more casual manner in which the correlated activation of a number of functional regions of interest constitutes a network. Having identified the putative neural nodes and observed their relation to the cognitive task, the assumption is made that they are meaningfully and functionally interconnected into a network that encodes the cognitive task. In fact, however, the functional interconnections between one node and others may be more speculative than empirical.

An alternative metaphor, as we have seen, is that these supposedly correlated nodes are simply locally enhanced parts of a widespread, if not almost universal, activation of the whole brain. As we learn more and more about the signal-to-noise relations of these brain responses, it is increasingly evident that there is a substantial amount of arbitrariness of what constitutes a "significant" center of activity—a "node." The point is that there are many ways to conceptualize the structure and functions of a brain network, not all of which might account for cognitively meaningful activity.

I now consider some criteria for acceptability of current macroneural network theories that specifically attempt to relate cognitive and neural activities. In pursing this goal, there are some types of theories that I deem to be of lesser relevance than the ones I consider here. Those excluded "network" theories are those that have little or no connection to the cognitive literature beyond a vague mention of analogous neural network-like properties. Thus, for example, much of the work carried out by the Artificial Intelligence (AI) or the Parallel Distributed Processing (PDP) communities has drifted far from the original heuristic of analyzing neuron-like networks. Both fields are nowadays constrained more by the properties and capabilities of computers than by the original impetus of driving discovery in cognitive neuroscience. Both fields are far from their neurophysiological roots, with nodes often consisting of high-level functions rather than entities with the physiological properties of neurons or brain centers. Although all of these approaches preserve some vestige of their neural roots in their language, most are no longer neurophysiologically relevant. None of this physiology-free work is targeted in this book. My interests are in those with joint cognitive and neural relevance; others will have to consider their mainly computational issues and constraints that characterize AI-type work. Although AI and PDP networks display some similarity with MCT networks (both types incorporate local nodes, interconnectivity, and parallelism) their neural content is vastly different; the one type operating exclusively at the behavioral level and the other incorporating that which we know about the biology of the brain. What the former can do for the latter is to develop some constraints on what mind-brain theories might eventually be like.

The Network Approach

In this chapter, I consider what progress has been made in developing specific psychobiological theories of mind-brain relations at the macroneural level—those that I have designated as MCT.

In principle, the experimental paradigm that should provide data supporting an MCT is relatively straightforward. There are two separate tasks in the development of such a theory. The first is the determination of supposed localized and relevant neural activity evoked by a particular cognitive task. The second is teasing out the properties of the interconnections between these locations in a way that makes interdisciplinary cognitive neuroscience theory even plausible. In other words, task the nervous system with some cognitive activity and determine the locations of the resulting brain responses and then infer the nature of the interconnecting pathways. This paradigm could in principle help us to gain some evidence, both functionally and structurally, of how multiple regions may interact. More often than not these days, this is done by means of an fMRI system. With luck and technical competence, the results should be reliable, provide robust evidence of discrete and demarcatable nodes and their interactions, and be both orderly and consistent enough to permit mathematical analysis. In practice, however, analyses of this kind are not likely to run so smoothly.

> A node or activation area is a localized peak of neural activity embodying the hypothesis that separable and distinct regions of the brain are activated by sufficiently well-defined cognitive processes. Functionally defined nodes may or may not agree with anatomically or architectonically defined areas.

What, then, are the components of a research protocol capable of elevating prototheories such as those discussed in Chapter 1 to an acceptable macroneural connectionist (i.e., network) theory of cognitive processes? The following list indicates the main steps that must be taken to develop a theory of the brain mechanisms of cognitive processes.

1. The psychological stimulus or task must be well defined and effectively controlled.
2. Whatever the physical stimulus or task directions, the cognitive response must be sufficiently stable so that it (i.e., the actual independent variable) will remain the same from trial to trial.

3. Brain responses must be also be reliable and consistent across methods and subject populations.[1]

4. A set of discrete and separable brain nodes (i.e., locations or activation sites) must be determined that is consistently and significantly associated with the cognitive task.

5. The functional connections between the nodes must either be empirically determined or inferable from the data. If inferred, the functional corrections must be shown at some point to correspond to anatomical connections. If there is any discrepancy and a comparable physical connection cannot eventually be found, the functional "connections" should not play any role in the development of a theory.

6. The directionality, valence, and trajectory of the valid interconnections must be established.

7. From these subtasks, we must then correlate, simulate, model, mimic, or encode the parameters of the psychological task to explain how brain leads to mind. This is, of course, the crux of the entire problem—demonstrating formally that, based on robust data, there is a reliable quantifiable or logical relation between the cognitive process and the brain response.

Ultimately, as the ideal test of such a theory, we would like to manipulate the state of the neural network and determine if the psychological state that generated the neural network activity can be regenerated. Only in this way can correlation be definitively established as causation. Unfortunately, such a manipulation of the brain components at either the macroneural or microneuronal level is almost never possible. In its place, we use less definitive criteria for choosing the best theory among possible alternatives or evaluating the fit of the theory to the data.

Goodness of fit by itself, however, is not itself a compelling argument for neuroreductionist theory development. Loose descriptive theories may be forced into compliance simply by adding another degree of freedom. Indeed, determination of what the theory cannot fit is a better test of a theory (Roberts & Pashler, 2000). Mere elegance or simplicity or even predictability is a greased slide to reifying what are essentially incorrect models. The real advantage of a mathematical model is that it serves as a plausibility test distinguishing between logical plausible and patently illogical models. The redundant and complex way in which the nervous system is constructed makes the use of Ockham's simplicity "razor" criterion inappropriate in cognitive neuroscience.

The Goal of MCT Theories

The first question with which we should deal with before discussing the details of several proposed theories is, what are the goals of MCT-type theories? In general, the answer to this rhetorical question is that it is to determine the location and nature of the mechanism or mechanisms by means of which brain activity is transmuted into cognitive activity. Ideally, this approach tries to map a particular set of cognitive processes onto a pattern of macroneural neural activation patterns. Maps of this kind are what Price and Friston (2005) and Poldrack (2006) referred to as "ontologies."[2] The linkage in the ontology should be strong enough so that in Price and Friston's words, "Function should predict structure and conversely structure should predict function" (p. 262). Price and Friston's and Poldrack's ontologies are closely associated with the localization assumption. In large part, they are maps of localized areas or lists of regions responding when the brain is active in a particular cognitive process. However, simply listing activated regions is a very limited step in the search for an explanation of the emergence of cognition from brain matter. To know where in the brain something is happening is not the same thing as knowing what is happening there.

The best that we could hope for, should the MCT approach be successful, is a statement of what parts of the brain seem to contain the neuronal mechanisms of mind and where they are located. In some special situations, mostly associated with sensory processes, it may be possible to find neural signals sufficiently correlated with transmitted information to permit us to determine the exact neural codes and to be able to recognize which sensory or perceptual process is currently underway. It must be emphasized, however, that this decoding of what transmissions and transformations are being executed (and this may only be possible in the sensory and motor domains) is not an explanation of the emergence of mental experience. A robust relation between the stimulus and neural response must initially be considered to be just a correlated "sign," not the psychoneural equivalent "code" of the cognition.

A sign is any neurophysiological signal that correlates with a cognitive process. A code is the actual neurophysiological action or mechanism (the psychoneural equivalent) that IS the cognitive process.

In practice, the identification of a sign is a reasonably plausible empirical goal—many such correlations may be observed. However, the task of establishing a true code for a cognitive process is not so simple and, arguably, may be impossible. One reason worth reemphasizing is Yule's classic admonition that correlation is not causation; and causation implies the identification of a code. Although there may be relatively high correlations between cognitive processes and macroneural responses gathered with fMRI systems, these responses are almost certainly signs and not codes. That is, they may be correlated activity driven by the stimulus but without any cognitive significance or psychoneural equivalence. In sum, not all correlated brain activity is ipso facto a code or psychoneural equivalent.

Despite these logical caveats, current theory development in cognitive neuroscience is now mainly driven by the metaphor of fMRI-specified, macroneural nodes interconnected by signal bearing tracts. Unfortunately, the ideal and strongest tests for psychoneural equivalence (i.e., a code as opposed to a sign) have rarely been carried out and then mainly in the sensory and motor systems. The difficulties in establishing psychoneural equivalence were made clear by the work of Martin et al. (2000).

What, then, would be the fulfillment of a neuroreductive MCT-type theory? Probably the clearest graphical presentation of an ideal version of an MCT theory is the one presented by Price and Friston (2005) in Figure 4.1.

The two domains of research (cognition and macroneural neurophysiology) shown here are related to each other, according to Price and Friston, by structure-function mappings. That is, according to this idealized model, for every identified cognitive process or subprocess there should be associated brain regions. For such an ideal model to exist, fulfillment of one criterion is absolutely necessary—there must be demonstrable and reliable empirical relationships between cognitive

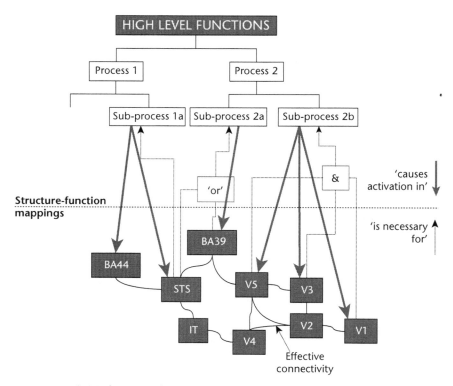

FIGURE 4.1 A Modern Ontology

(From Price and Friston, 2005, with the permission of the publisher)

modules and brain locations. A major problem with this idealized MCT model, however, is that true equivalence may be a fluctuating pattern of responses between multiple brain locations and several overlapping cognitive processes. In that case, a dynamic and complex system may be a better metaphor for mind-brain correspondence than any unique one-to-one relations. This kind of four-dimensional stability may be very elusive, indeed.

To actually produce this idealized kind of mapping, two different kinds of experiments must be carried out. The first is the prototypical paradigm of evoking a cognitive state by appropriate instructions or stimuli and then determining which regions of the brain are reliably activated. The second kind of experiment, which is designed to validate the structure-function mapping by showing that it produces the original cognitive state when the set of brain regions is activated, is much more difficult, if not impossible, to carry out. The reason for this is obvious; we do not have the kind of control over the activities of brain regions to actually establish the *necessity* of some pattern of neural activity in the manner proposed by Martin et al. (2000). To produce the same pattern of activation as that generated by a stimulus in order to reproduce the original cognitive process is a task not yet achieved at either the microneuronal or macroneural level. Without the anchor of empirical evidence from this second part of the task—to establish the necessity of a particular configuration of nodes—we can rarely be sure that the recorded brain responses are directly associated with the cognitive processes or are just irrelevant, albeit, correlated signals—signs.

Achieving the goals of MCT theories, of course, becomes extremely challenging if localized, demarcatable activation peaks or nodes do not exist. That indeed is the suggestion of the recent work of Thyreau et al. (2012) and Gonzalez-Castillo et al. (2012); research that will be considered in Chapter 5.

4.2 Qualitative MCT Theories

Theories, as we have seen so far, come in many varieties—verbal, behavioral simulations, formal mathematical, and pictorial. In this section, I survey a number of the most prominent presentations that describe possible arrangements of neural-cognitive systems that may be considered to be qualitative; that is, not involving quantitative system analyses.

Mesulam's Pioneering Distributed Cognitive Theory for Directed Attention

As noted in Chapter 1, the notion of interconnected networks of macroneural nodes of activity has been around for many years. (The classic example is Papez's MCT of emotions, 1937.) One of the first to apply the concept of networks of macroneural brain regions in the modern brain imaging era was Mesulam (1990). Influenced to a substantial degree by the concepts of parallel distribution championed by Rumelhart and McClelland (1986) and McClelland and Rumelhart (1986),[3] Mesulam suggested specific neural network models for attention, language, and memory.

It is interesting to note which brain areas or "nodes" are incorporated into Mesulam's pioneering MCT. He included the superior colliculus, frontal eye fields, intraparietal sulcus, medial parietal cortex, superior parietal lobe, superior temporal sulcus, the cingulate, the reticular activating system, and, in addition, parts of Brodmann areas 45, 46, and 6. In addition, specific connections are diagrammed between these nodes. Therefore, Mesulam's MCT was a specific model of a network of particular macroneural regions of the brain that he believed operated as an interactive system to instantiate the cognitive process we call directed attention.

Although we have now gone far beyond the details of this early theory, Mesulam's approach was very much in the spirit of more recent MCTs. Based on what was then the best available research and clinical evidence at the time, his model included all of the elements—nodes, connections, and other mechanisms—that characterize modern theories. Feedback, feed forward, and lateral connections are all present, as are multiply interconnected nodes. Mesulam's most important contribution, however, was his organization of these parts into an integrated, albeit hypothetical, system in which all the parts necessarily contributed to the function of the whole system but in which the whole system was necessary to carry out the intended cognitive process of directing the subject's attention. In particular, he argued that the disruption of any connection or that damage to any of the anatomical components of the system would disrupt some part of its overall cognitive function. Focus on the whole system, therefore, became primary, not the function of any individual component. This metaphor is still the main conceptual foundation of macroneural brain organization (and, thus, of cognitive organization) today. Mesulam was also one of the first to point out that, because of the complexity of interactions, there could be paradoxical responses in which the reduction of a stimulus could actually increase the brain response. Thus, Mesulam implicitly introduced the idea of disinhibition into MCT discussions.

In sum, Mesulam was also among the early modern workers to introduce the important idea of a collection of specific anatomical structures working together in a complex interactive network to collectively represent a particular cognitive process.[4]

Alternative Qualitative MCT Theories of Directed Attention

The decades that have passed since Mesulam's pioneering work have changed the details of his proposed neural network theory, but many of the general principles he described remain germane to current theory. For example, Bundesen et al. (2005) developed a theory of visual attention and proposed an MCT that could embody it. In doing so, they made a very important additional point—their theory (and all other similar versions of MCT theories) "does not depend critically on a particular anatomical localization of the proposed computation" (p. 295). By this, I believe they meant that the nodes in their MCT were not specifically localized in the brain. Thus, function need not map directly onto specific brain regions; instead the nodes could be themselves distributed processes, a suggestion that is recurring ever more frequently these days. It also reminds us that many different MCT neuroanatomical networks can fit the same data. There is no a priori reason to assume that any one of these network models is any more correct than any other. However, Bundesen et al. did offer up a specific neural model of visual attention based on newer developments in neurophysiology and neuroanatomy than were available to Mesulam.

Another model of an attention system has been proposed by Posner, Sheese, Odludas, and Tang (2006). In Posner et al.'s theory, the anterior cingulate is proposed as the core of an attention system. Though it may differ from the other two theories of attention in anatomic detail, the characteristic properties of an MCT are present—multiple interconnected nodes and directed functional interconnections.

A useful exercise to illustrate the lack of convergence onto a single theory is to compare the regions invoked in the three theories.

Mesulam

Subcortical

- Reticular Activating System
- Pulvinar
- Superior Colliculus

Cortical (Sample)

- Cingulate
- Frontal Eye Fields
- Parietal Cortex
- Temporal Cortex
- Parts of Brodmann areas 45, 46, and 6

Bundesen, Habekost, and Kyllingsbaek

Subcortical

- Pulvinar
- Lateral Geniculate
- Thalamic Reticular Nucleus

Cortical

* Occipital Regions (in general)

Posner, Sheese, Odludas, and Tang

Cortical

* BA 22—Temporal parietal junction
* BA 7—Superior parietal gyrus
* BA 6 and 10—Frontal lobe

There are great differences between these three lists that make it impossible to make an exact comparison of these three MCTs of attention; each was based on slightly different kinds of cognitive tasks that probably produced different results for each of the different methods. Furthermore, each group of investigators presented their model in a slightly different pictorial manner. Most of all, the psychological language they used to define attention was probably different from one of these studies to another. Nevertheless, it is clear that there are substantial differences between the three MCT theories with regard to brain regions supposedly involved in the cognitive process we call "visual attention." The reasons for these discrepancies are certainly plentiful, but at least include, psychological language, cognitive experimental designs, technical methodologies, statistical methods, and, perhaps, most of all, the preconceptions that investigators had about what they expected to see.

Other Qualitative Macroneural Connectionist Theories of Cognitive Processes

A number of other MCT-type theories have been proposed over the years. Often these are intentionally limited to a subset of what are considered to be the most salient of the responding brain areas. Thus, for example, in his quest to analyze changes in brain organization during a semantic processing task, McIntosh (2000) abstracted, from what must be a much more complex network, a simple model of brain area activations under three modes of responding. The respective PET images were then analyzed to show the nature of the interconnections between a group of responding Brodmann areas and how they differed for three types of responses—a computer mouse click, a spoken response, and simply thinking.

McIntosh's model is particularly interesting for several reasons. First, it was developed relatively early in the development of the MCT concept. Unlike the purely anatomical charts (e.g., Kaas, 2004; Van Essen et al., 1992) that mainly characterized this epoch, it included not only the valence but also the relative magnitude of the strength of the interconnections.

Another MCT emphasizing the strength and directionality of the interconnections was proposed by Friston and Price (2011) in which a comparison was made between reading and object naming.

These two MCTs (Friston & Price, 2011; McIntosh, 2000) have some common features that help us to understand what can be expected from this theoretical approach. First, they identified specific regions of the brain (putative nodes) that seem to be differentially involved in tasks that are distinguished by some aspect of the cognitive or response process. Second, they identified functional interconnections that may not be obvious in the raw anatomical data. Third, they assigned relative effectiveness and direction to these interconnecting links. These three properties are now assumed to be necessary features of any MCT theory of cognition.

An Alternative Data Presentation

In most of the MCT-type theories discussed so far, the standard means of displaying findings is in the form of a "block diagram" in which the blocks identified the involved neural components and interconnecting lines identified the presumed courses of the neural tracts that might connect the blocks. It is a truism that the way that data are presented can force our thinking into a particular mode. Thus, it seems plausible to suggest that different modes of plotting data from an experiment may themselves lead to alternative theoretical conclusions. This is what seems to be happening as evidenced in a comprehensive meta-analysis of the literature concerning the neural basis of emotion reported by Lindquist et al. (2012). In this article, they provided an alternative means of presenting the complex array of data associating emotion with particular brain regions and concluded something quite different from that inferred from other kinds of data displays. Their presentation was based on a logistic regression[5] in which the probability that a particular cognitive process would activate a particular brain region was represented on a polar coordinate plot. In this novel presentation, shown in Figure 4.2, the length of the radii indicated the deviations between resting and activation scores during emotional cognitive activities. The smaller concentric circles (with negative values) indicated the probability that there would *not be an increase* in neural activity associated with emotion compared to a measurement during rest. The values represented by the larger of the concentric circles (with positive values) indicated the probability that there *would be an increase* in the activity of particular brain regions associated with a particular cognitive activity.

The main theoretical conclusion arrived at by Lindquist et al. (2012) from this kind of presentation was that there are no specific brain regions that encode an emotion such as fear, anger, sadness, or disgust. They, thus, rejected the dominant "locationist" and function-specific theory of cognitive and brain modularity. In its place, their meta-analysis suggested that there was a variety

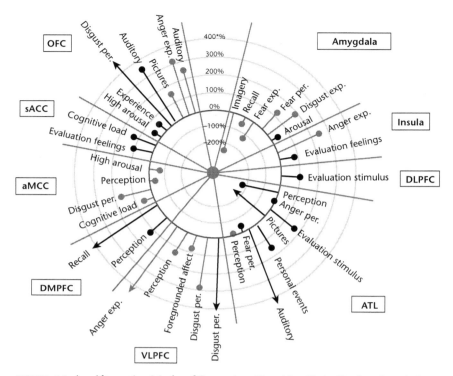

FIGURE 4.2 An Alternative Mode of Presenting Cognitive Brain Region Associations (From Lindquist et al., 2012 with the permission of the publisher.)

of brain regions associated with any one of these emotional experiences. Rather than a specific site or a small group of sites being the equivalent of a particular emotional experience, their meta-analysis, as embodied in Figure 4.2, led them to argue strongly for the idea of a differential pattern of what may be many of the same brain regions being associated with different kinds of emotions. They, thus, distinguish between the function-specific, locationist approach and

> the psychological constructionist approach (i.e., the hypothesis that discrete emotion categories are constructed of more general brain networks not specific to those categories) . . . A set of interacting brain regions commonly involved in basic psychological operations of both an emotional and non-emotional nature are active during emotion experience and perception across a range of discrete emotion categories.
>
> *(p. 121)*

Lindquist and her colleagues make important points that speak to the future of cognitive neuroscience. Not the least of these is that there are no specific locations for the representation of cognitive processes. However, even more important is the implication that it may be the pattern of activity across major portions of the brain that is the foundation of the neural representation of cognitive processes.

The general point made by all of the MCT models of brain-cognitive relationships discussed so far is that the brain represents cognition by patterns of activation in multiple regions of the brain. However these data are plotted, the idea is that different parts of the brain work together to produce cognition. A corollary is that these regions are interconnected by neural tracts of variable direction, valence, and effectiveness. From one point of view, this is a step forward from the original concept of unique function-specific regions that originally populated mind-brain theories. Unfortunately, none of them are sufficiently quantitative to permit evaluative testing. The best they can do is to qualitatively emphasize the distributed nature of the brain responses. This is an important step, but a more specific evaluation of MCT depends on more quantitative approaches to theory. This is the purpose of the next section of this chapter.

4.3   Quantitative MCT Theories

In this section, I examine in detail two recent formal mathematical MCTs in order to further gauge progress, to add to our understanding of the method, and to determine the state of the most advanced MCT theories in this field. The exemplar research articles I have chosen to discuss are, first, a very recent study reported by Schroll, Vitay, and Hamker (2012) and, second, the somewhat older work of Ashby et al. (2007). Both theories are empowered by mathematical models that represent a major step forward from the essentially qualitative or pictorial representations characteristic of the qualitative theories discussed earlier in this chapter. I have chosen them because they are among the most comprehensive examples of well-studied and important cognitive processes—in the first case, working memory and response selection, and in the second, perceptual categorization. Both MCT approaches are based on multiple nodes and heavy interconnections among many regions of the brain. Both theories involve both cortical and subcortical mechanisms. Although less emphasis is placed on cortical mechanisms than I would have preferred in either study, the general principles underlying regional interactions remain the same. Both theories are also notable in being relatively complete in terms of supporting empirical evidence. Most important, both incorporate mathematical tests of their logical plausibility evaluated by computational simulations, something that is missing in the primarily qualitative MCTs of the previous sections.

A Quantitative MCT Theory of Working Memory and Response Selection

In this section, I consider in detail the quantitative neural theory of working memory and response selection developed by Schroll et al. (2012). As noted, this is not the first attempt to develop a formal neural theory of working memory. A pioneering precursor of this model is the work of Baddeley (2003) in which he summarized both his psychological[6] and neurophysiological postulates.

Despite the number of theories of working memory, work in this field is, as usual, complicated by the fact that slight deviations in stimulus design or subject samples can often produce great differences in both the evoked brain images and the behavioral responses. For example, differences between what are defined by their investigators as spatial and object working memory are reputed to activate different brain regions (e.g., see Smith & Jonides, 1999).

Beyond the almost universal association of working memory (and all other cognitive processes) with the prefrontal cortex, there is little agreement on which other parts of the brain are involved.[7] Emphasis has been placed on the cortical components but, as we now see, other researchers have emphasized the role of subcortical components of the brain.

I have chosen to consider Schroll et al.'s (2012) work in detail because it represents an up-to-date and comprehensive quantitative approach to MCT theory whose methods and concepts are spelled out in relatively complete detail. First, however, it is necessary to make clear exactly what the Schroll et al. model is. In their words, it is a connectionist theory of how a network of "parallel and hierarchically interconnected loops provides a potential anatomic substrate for both [working memory] WM processes and response selection" (p. 59). Like all MCT theories, it operates at the level of macroneural units of the brain and dotes on the directed connections between the various centers and regions of the brain. It is unusual in testing the plausibility of its conclusions with a computer simulation of a mathematical model. In this regard, it is a fine example of what an MCT is supposed to be. Thus, it is well placed to serve as one prototype for our discussion of advantages, disadvantages, and conceptual properties of this type of theorizing. Figure 4.3 is Schroll et al.'s proposed architecture.

However complex this network may seem to be, as the authors pointed out, it is certainly only a part of a much more diverse and inclusive network of brain regions involved in working memory. Although this model incorporates two regional loops of brain components presumably underlying the specified cognitive processes (the prefrontal-basal ganglia-thalamic loop mainly on the left side and the motor cortex-thalamic-putamen loop primarily on the right side of Figure 4.3), it is not and probably cannot be assumed to be complete given the current state of our technology. Schroll et al. (2012) explicitly pointed out that there are a number of other brain regions that are also thought to be involved in working memory and response selection that are not incorporated in their

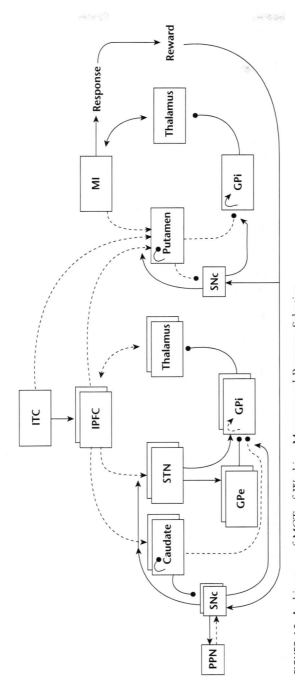

FIGURE 4.3 Architecture of MCT of Working Memory and Response Selection

(From Schroll, Vitay, & Hamker, 2012, with the permission of the publisher)

model. These include a "direct basal ganglia pathway" and a "hyperdirect pathway of the motor loop."

A centrally important aspect of their model is the neurophysiological evidence that led not only to the inclusion of these anatomically defined macroregions but also to the properties of the interconnections between them. Schroll and his colleagues were specific in answering the question, why were particular regions chosen from among the many that might be involved in working memory or response selection as components of the architecture of this model? Their answer to this question is that the role of virtually every component of their model is justified by some kind of physiological or functional evidence. This includes not only the specification of the various interconnections, but also their valence, direction, and relative influence. For example, the involvement of the lateral prefrontal cortex in their representation of working memory was specifically based on the work of Owen et al. (1999) who was one of the first to have suggested an association of this region with working memory.

Other subcortical components of this model are justified by similar extrapolations of what were believed to be known anatomy or physiology. The caudate nucleus, a part of the striatum, for example, is known to be negatively correlated with progress in reward related learning, an observation attributed to Delgado, Miller, Inati, and Phelps (2005) among others. Thalamic nuclei are incorporated into the model in large part for their reported ability to modify behavior when stimulated or lesioned.

Similarly, the inhibitory or excitatory effect of anatomically or functionally known interconnections suggested their valence. The nature of these interactions was then linked to particular transmitter substances used at synapses. For example, according to Schroll and his colleagues (2012), the pedunculopontine nucleus in the brainstem (a region associated with many cognitive processes by Winn, 2006) had been shown to send out cholinergic fibers that "recruit quiescent dopamine neurons" (Di Giovanni & Shi, 2009, p. 673).[8]

Hopefully, this discussion of Schroll et al.'s work provides some insight to the selection process and, perhaps even more important, into the kinds of decisions that had to be made in the preparation of their MCT. Whatever its limitations, one is hard pressed to find a more complete example of a quantitative MCT. Perhaps the most important aspect of Schroll and his colleagues' work is that they programmed a mathematical model allowing them to carry out a formal test of their theory. This is a very important step in theory development of this kind because mathematics permits us to test the plausibility of its fundamental logic and basic postulates. Without such a mathematical analysis, the aggregation of all of the supporting evidence into the pictorial model depicted in Figure 4.3 would be more akin to the kind of verbal obfuscation or conceptual hand waving that characterizes so much of purely qualitative neural network "theories."

My current goal is to illustrate their theory's general organization, emphasize the concepts that underlay its accomplishments, and evaluate the degree to which it approximates macroneural findings. The formulation offered by these investigators was a system of differential equations. Each anatomical part (e.g., thalamus, caudate) of the model was represented by a couple of equations that were also intended to describe the membrane potentials and the firing rates of simulated "neurons" in that region. The equations for each brain region's membrane potential and firing rate are linked to all of the others by common terms in the set of differential equations representing the system.

Before going further, it is important to point out that in my opinion this insertion of the terminology of membrane potentials and firing rates—properties of individual neurons—is a manipulation that is neither necessary nor justified by the authors.[9] Because their model is formulated in terms of data for macroneural brain regions and their functions, these microneuronal terms can, at best, only be surrogates for what are really the macroneural "responses" of regions such as the thalamus. This is an interesting point, because it once again emphasizes the admonition that the terms of the mathematical equations are neutral with regard to underlying mechanisms. In this case, for example, the same mathematics was equally capable of describing the functions of membranes and neurons and the macroneural responses regions of the brain.

An MCT Theory of Perceptual Categorization

The second example of a modern, fully developed MCT representative of the current state of the art to be considered here is one proposed by Ashby et al. (2007). Their goal was to develop a "neurobiological" theory of "how categorization judgments become automatic in tasks that depend on procedural learning" (p. 632). Once again, they were dealing with a well-known cognitive process that had a substantial amount of empirical psychological research supporting the details of their model.

The key neurobiological point made by Ashby and his colleagues was that there is a transition between the brain mechanisms accounting for inexpert and effortful categorization to those serving the automatic, well-, or over-learned version of the process. They speculated that the process of learning to categorize objects should, therefore, show some kind of a transfer of localization from the prefrontal cortex to other, mostly subcortical, regions as the degree of automaticity increases. The functional distinction being made is that prior to automatic categorization, the process is more akin to working memory; afterwards, it is more like procedural learning or other forms of implicit learning; that is, learning without any specific instructions or even awareness on the part of the subject.

The formal theory proposed Ashby et al. is designed to show how these functional and neural shifts might occur. A diagram of the model they built is shown in Figure 4.4. Of course, as in the Schroll et al. (2012) theory, all of these investigators acknowledge this must be a very incomplete statement of the full range of brain components that are actually involved in a cognitive process such

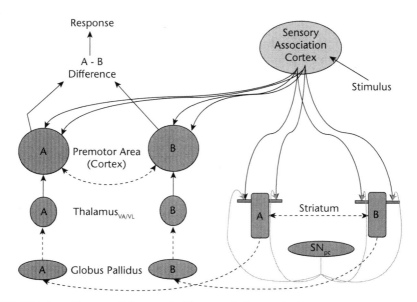

FIGURE 4.4 A Theory of Automatic Perceptual Categorization

(From Ashby, Ennis, & Spiering, 2007, with the permission of the publisher)

as perceptual categorization. However, Ashby and his colleagues argue that these are the main regions that have some sort of empirical evidence for their involvement in categorization.

Ashby and Maddox (2005) also documented a substantial amount of supportive evidence behind their model, specifically highlighting fMRI-based associations (Nomura et al., 2007) drawn between rule-based learning (a form of working memory) and both frontal and temporal activity, on the one hand, and "information-integration learning" (a form of implicit learning) and the subcortical caudate nucleus, on the other hand. As usual, there is some inconsistency in the data. For example, Ashby and his colleagues allude to single cell recording studies (e.g., Freedman, Riesenhuber, Poggio, & Miller, 2003) that do not support the clear-cut separation of working memory–type activity in the cerebrum and implicit learning-type activity subcortically. These inconsistencies and controversial views are not unexpected given the difference in technologies and procedures used in the different types of research they cited.

Ashby et al. (2007) went on to also introduce what they consider to be supportive data from the neurophysiology and neurochemistry of single neurons. In particular, they mention dopamine, glutamate, and GABA transmitter substances as playing an important role in their model. Once again, as in the Schroll et al. (2012) theory, it appears that the mathematical model makes minimum use of this information, mainly in determining the excitatory or inhibitory valence of particular tracts.

Also like the Schroll et al. theory, the formal computerization of the Ashby et al. model is based on a system of interacting differential equations. These equations represent properties of the network such as "activation" in the responses of a sensory cortical or striatal "unit." Although there remains some ambiguity concerning what a "unit" is, in fact, the specific meaning is not terribly consequential in this type of model, the mathematical model being able to represent macro or microneuronal components. In sum, Ashby et al. have developed a computational model of automatic categorization based on a variety of psychological, neurophysiological, and neuroanatomical evidence. They have used this empirical support to develop a system of differential equations that is capable of simulating a number of brain processes by fitting these equations to behavioral data.

Evaluation of the Two Quantitative Theories

A necessary preliminary step in any evaluation of models such as those proposed by Schroll et al. (2012) and by Ashby et al. (2007) is to establish what they were trying to accomplish in the development of their respective theories. The goal in the first of these studies was to test whether an arrangement of neuroanatomical nodes could simulate the cognitive process of working memory and response selection. Specifically, Schroll (2012) and his colleagues stated that they were trying to

> present a biologically meaningful computational model of how these [cortico-basalganglio-thalamic] loops contribute to the organization of working memory and the development of response behavior.
>
> *(p. 59)*

The context in which they develop their model is a macroneural one. The grounding assumption is that the interaction of a system of nodes (i.e., functionally defined brain regions) identified from previous research can be associated with the aforementioned cognitive processes. Clearly, this is a theory in which the macroneural interactions between brain regions are the salient events.

The goals of the work of Ashby and his colleagues (2007) are also clear-cut. They state,

> A biologically detailed computational model is described of how categorization judgments become automatic in tasks that depend on procedural learning. The model assumes two neural pathways from sensory association cortex to the premotor area that mediates response selection. A longer and slower path projects to the premotor area via the striatum, Globus pallidus, and thalamus. A faster, purely cortical path projects directly to the premotor areas.
>
> *(p. 632)*

The detailed discussions of these two contributions were carried out to provide some good examples of the current status of modern MCT theories of cognition. Their strong points include the following:

1. The theories are founded on a strong base of psychological evidence and involve relatively well-defined cognitive processes.
2. There is a presumptive empirical argument for each and every component shown in their respective flowchart-type models. The selection of the various anatomical nodes and connecting tracts in each case is also based on what they believe is robust empirical evidence from neuroanatomical and neurophysiological investigations associated with cognitive processes.
3. Hypothetical, but clear, pictorial and mathematical representations are made of the manner in which specific areas interconnected with other specific areas.
4. The theories are formalized by establishing mathematical models that are presumed to simulate the functions of the various units and their interactions.
5. When the computational versions of each theory are run, they are shown to mimic or simulate some measures of the associated behavior.
6. In general, the approach taken in both of these theories, like all mathematical models, constrains otherwise verbal explanations to logically and deductively test events and transformations for plausibility. Implausible and inconsistent hand waving or verbal imprecisions are minimized by this approach. The formal mathematical model embodied in each of these two theories establishes the *sufficiency* of each theory as a putative neuroreductive explanation of the cognitive processes being studied. This is a major advantage of this approach; at the very least, it is able to provide a possible and plausible neuroreductive description of a complex process that seems to simulate cognitive processing.

On the other hand, the MCT approach to theory making taken by both of these theories has a number of limitations, including the following:

1. The fundamental postulate of the theory is that the respective cognitive pro-, cesses are encoded by macroneural mechanisms. However, current thinking suggests that a microneuronal approach may be more likely for reasons of basic principle.
2. Their respective selection of the nodes and connecting tracts is necessarily based on incomplete empirical evidence. The system is obviously very much more complicated than the abstractions represented by these two studies. Indeed, there is an increasing possibility that many more parts of the brain (even the whole brain) than just those modeled are involved in any cognitive process. Therefore, it is impossible to assure that all relevant nodes and interconnections are incorporated into the postulates and deductions of the proposed theories. This is a serious imitation because the addition or subtraction of one node may drastically change the performance of the entire system. As

a result, theories of this kind are at best just sufficient, can never be necessary, and are always susceptible to the vagaries of new evidence.

3. The empirical data on which these theories are based are nowhere as robust as is suggested by their respective citations. Variability and inconsistency are typical throughout this field; controversy regarding the most basic points is constant.

4. The two-dimensional depiction of these theories may obscure the three-dimensional nature of the network adding a further note of complexity to this kind of theory building that is often overlooked.

5. The two mathematical models required some additional manipulation (e.g., shaping or tweaking) of the mathematical equations that had not been included in the original theories to make the model's response fit the empirical data.

6. There were inadequately justified transitions from macroneural to micro-neuronal languages in both theories. Whereas the basic assumptions of the model, as well as the model itself, were phrased almost entirely in terms of macroneural nodes and tracts, the measured output of the model was often translated to the language of membrane potentials or neuronal firing rates (or both). This vocabulary conversion serves no obvious function and confuses the particulars of the respective theories.

7. A major handicap of mathematical theories such as the two reviewed here is that they are not able to establish the unique necessity of their particular theoretical instantiations. No matter how well the responses of the models "fit" the original behavioral observations, it is clear that these two models are not unique or *necessary* answers to the question of how cognition or behavior emerges from network interactions. Other theoretical approaches organized in different ways, both mathematically and anatomically, may be able to simulate the target behavior equally well. In other words, these models describe possible, plausible, or sufficient mechanisms of their respective behaviors, but do not authenticate them as the necessary ones actually being executed by the brain. Obviously, this is not a limitation solely of cognitive neuroscience—it is a universal problem faced by all sciences.

In sum, though limited and incomplete, this type of mathematical "theory" is about the best we have in the domain of macroneural theories.

4.4 Graph Theory

The two theories evaluated in the previous section use conventional mathematical methods (differential equations) to develop a model of interactions among a number of macroneural nodes. An alternative approach—graph theory—uses quite a different kind of mathematics to describe the organization of a complex network of nodes and their interconnections. Before discussing this formulation, it is important to note that a graph theory model has quite a different goal than do the ones based on the analytic equations (differential equations) just described. The analytic methods just discussed were specifically designed to describe or predict the *behavior* of the modeled system. They constituted a functional simulation seeking to show how a network behaved or functioned when the properties of the "nodes" and "edges" were controlled or how neurophysiological observations might participate in network functions.

> A graph is a means of representing the network structure of a complex system in which nodes (vertices) are interconnected by connecting links (edges). It is primarily a means of describing the static organization of the network.

An alternative approach, represented by graph theory, concentrates not on the *functional* properties of the network but on its structural properties; that is, on the organization and arrangement of the nodes and edges and what these structural factors could tell us about the properties of the network. Rather than attempting to describe how a relatively simple network might function, this alternative provides a means of representing the *structural properties* of networks in general.

Graph theory, since its reinvention by Harary (1969), has found many applications in many different sciences. Many of these applications have to do with the plausibility or proof of theorems of the structural constraints operating on a particular kind of graph. Graphs have also been used to describe molecular and atomic structures and can distinguish between plausible and impossible network configurations within which some things can be done whereas others are impossible.

Recently, graph theory, now considered to be a branch of topology, has been applied to characterizing the properties of neural networks. Although a graph theoretical explanation can describe only the properties of a network like the brain (it is unlikely that the mind-brain problem would be solved using this approach), it can provide valuable information about the possible organization of the networks of the brain (Bullmore & Sporns, 2009).

In a very useful tutorial, Wang et al. (2010) describes some of the measures or properties of neuronal graphs that might potentially help us characterize the organization of the brain. Among the most notable to which they direct our attention are as follows:

1. The *degree* of a graph is the number of edges linked to it.
2. The mean value of the degrees of all nodes in a network is a measure of the *connectivity* of the network.
3. Network *efficiency* is defined as the ratio of the number of existing edges to the number of all possible edges.

4. There are several kinds of nodal *centrality*, but one kind is encapsulated as the average distance from a node to all others in the network.
5. Of special interest to neuroscientists is the idea of *modularity*. Modularity is defined as a clustering of nodes such that the interconnections among them are stronger than the interconnections with distant nodes.
6. *Hierarchy* is indicated by the number of nodes that are connected to other nodes that are not connected to each other.

(Paraphrased from Wang et al., 2010)

To the degree that nodes are real and that it is possible to measure these network properties, they may be used as indicators of the organization of the brain, perhaps even as a measure of brain changes in learning to the degree that learning changes the structural organization of the brain. Wang et al., for example, applied these measures to the study of resting state fMRI and suggested possible applications to problems of psychopathology.

In general, however, many applications of graph theory are actually better representations of the anatomic rather than the functional aspects of the network (e.g., Iturria-Medina, Sotero, Canales-Rodriguez, Aleman-Gomez, & Melie-Garcia, 2008). This can be useful in determining the organizational nature of the network, but by itself, it does not provide insight into the cognitively germane issues beyond the generalities of network-like structures of which the brain is indisputatively a prime example.

The graph theory approach to understanding the organization of the brain is far easier to describe than it is to apply. However easy it may be to carry out the simple calculations that allow us to provide a numerical score for a property such as "centrality," it is far harder to accumulate the empirical data that characterize a realistic neural network in the variable and inconstant environment defined by brain imaging equipment.

4.5 Multivariate Analysis

It now appears that we may be in the midst of a transition to an even newer mind-brain metaphor based on multivariate pattern analysis. This new concept of brain organization is based on the idea that cognitive processes are encoded by a multitude of relatively small (compared with the blocks of an MCT theory) active regions that are spread widely (and irregularly) around the brain. The basic idea is that it is not a particular place or a localized activation area of the brain, or even a specific cluster of nodes, but rather a *pattern* of activity encoded by many small neural entities, not yet at the microneuronal level of individual neurons, but at the limits of voxel resolution level of current MRI systems. The reduction of the size of the salient activation region (i.e., the voxel) is a step towards theories formulated at the microneuronal scale at which the neurons and their interactions must be studied if we are to understand the neural basis of cognition. Although we may arrive at that level someday, it is likely that the numerousness and size of the neurons in even a minimally cognitively significant network would still preclude solution of the general mind-brain problem in the near future.

> A voxel is the smallest three-dimensional volume (analogous to a two-dimensional pixel) whose size is defined by the resolving power of the instrument being used. Except for a few special situations, the minimum practical voxel size of an fMRI system is still too large to measure neurons. Thus the best currently available MRI system still operates at a fairly gross level that encompasses thousands, if not millions, of neurons.

As a result of the increasing corpus of data showing widely dispersed and multiply responsive brain regions to a cognitive task, mathematical techniques referred to generically as Multi-Voxel Pattern Analysis or Multi-Variate Pattern Analysis (MVPA in either case) have begun to be applied to represent the distributed information from fMRI experiments. These techniques are designed to provide a quantitative foundation for what is essentially a multiplicity of salient data values whose individual roles in the pattern may not be fixed but whose collective operation may be salient. In this regard, they differ from most of the earlier studies in which a single discriminating parameter was used to distinguish between two states—most notably control and experimental conditions. No longer is a simple difference between two (or a few) responses considered to be an adequate measure of relevant brain activity; instead, with a MVPA, differences in the overall pattern of many responses are assumed collectively to describe the overall state of the system.

As Haxby (2010) pointed out, the use of MVPA leads to a different metaphor for the brain's organization than that invoked in previous models. Stimulated by this new approach, he suggested that we should now tend to think in the following terms:

> A brain area has the capacity to represent a variety of stimuli or cognitive states, Local variation of response strength within a brain area is a signal that reflects changes in representational state.
>
> Weak activity, as well as strong activity, can be important in specifying the representational state of a brain area.

> *(p. 57)*

To his suggestions, we can also add another—because it is the pattern of many activations and not the details of any one, the same cognitive process may be encoded by what may initially appear to be different patterns at different times; the behavior of each element of the pattern being more or less inconsequential. In one instance, a given voxel may be activated but, in another functionally equivalent pattern, it may not participate or actually be reduced compared to its resting level of activity. In other instances, a voxel may be activated not because the cognitive task used as an independent variable is driving it but because of some irrelevant second order effect. By looking at a pattern of activity, rather than individual components, some overall stability may be introduced even if localized responses remain highly variable. Perhaps even more important, MVPA suggests a new metaphor for mind-brain relations that was not implicit in previous MCT theories—one of flexibility, variability, and momentary inconsistency of the neural response. This is a major change in our thinking from the constant role played by the blocks in an MCT-type theory.

The key idea in the application of the MVPA method, therefore, is that no single unit or component or particular group of units and components is definitive in encoding a cognitive process; instead, it is the overall pattern of a distributed response that is critical. This is far more biologically plausible, given the distributed nature of brain responses and their variability, than is the traditional metaphor of localized, function-specific nodes.

There are several steps in the application of MVPA depending on one's goals. The first step in any case is to carry out imaging work to identify the smallest possible voxels associated with a cognitive process. These voxels may be a large group, not all of which are going to be representative codes from trial to trial. To reiterate, the idea behind the MVPA is that a pattern may consist of a different set of participating voxels from trial to trial. It is the overall pattern that matters, not the particular constituent voxels.

Nor do the participating voxels necessarily have to be limited to those that are responding at a level significantly *above* chance—the absence or reduction of activity in a particular voxel may be a key indication of cognitive activity. Obviously, not all responsive voxels are specifically involved in the cognitive process under study. Some may be activated by uncontrolled variables, and some may simply be statistical anomalies. Nevertheless, the pattern is presumed to collectively represent a coordinated set of response values that, it is hoped, will be differentially and distinctively related to different cognitive tasks in some orderly way. This first step is primarily an empirical task.

Following the identification of a significant and reliable pattern of responding voxels, a second step is to determine not just which voxels are responding in a correlated manner but also what is the distinctive pattern of these voxels for particular cognitive processes. This is accomplished by applying more or less standard multidimensional analysis techniques. For example, the Princeton MVPA program package to carry out this operation can be found at http://code.google.com/p/princeton-mvpa-toolbox/.

A third step involves some form of preliminary testing with known stimuli to train the pattern analyzer to distinctively respond to a specific cognitive response. Such a training step is useful if the experimenter's goal is to establish a connection between a particular multivariate brain and a cognitive state in order that the distinctive brain state for that cognitive state can be subsequently recognized.

The overall pattern of neural activity identified by multidimensional pattern recognizers associated with a particular cognitive process is a multidimensional vector in which both the number and pattern of responding voxels presumably encode the cognitive process. The essential aspect of these vectors is that the location and function of each of the various components may be not only variable but also unknown. No longer are we searching for specific localized brain regions associated with particular functions; instead, the goal is to identify a pattern of response of voxels, parts of a distributed system, that maintain a particular pattern of relationships to each other. There is, therefore, no need to attribute a particular fixed function to any one of the significant voxels. It is the relation of all of the responsive voxels to each other that is the key to cognitive representation. This relationship may vary from one trial or subject to another while still preserving the essential pattern of information.

In many ways, MVPA is an important conceptual leap forward; it represents another step away from the notion of fixed locale and function-specific that has been inherent in earlier work since the heyday of phrenology and that still permeates brain imaging research. Fixed regional activations, whether they are isolated or components in a network, no longer are restricted to instantiating particular cognitive functions. Indeed, given the variability of responses at all levels of the analysis, the flexibility of individual areas of the brain to participate in the representation of multiple cognitive processes becomes increasingly apparent. Similarly, the variability and adaptability of the brain in using different patterns of neural activity to represent a particular cognitive process become increasingly tenable.

MVPA is influential, therefore, in carrying us forward towards a revised metaphor of the brain that may be much closer to the reality of the way in which the brain encodes mental activity. It approaches the scale of the microneuronal pattern of activity in networks of individual neurons—but it is still not at that level. However, we are no longer restricted to Brodmann-sized chunks of the brain or the proposed functional-specificity of specific activation regions determined by fMRI systems. In its place, we are now conceptualizing a brain that is made up of relatively small, widely distributed, interacting, and, most important, transitory, interacting units. The two metaphors—the one underlying multifactorial pattern analysis and the Hebb hypothesis—are, at least, approaching each other's scale.[10]

There are several additional points to be considered. First, MVPA is no more a theoretical panacea towards unraveling the mind-brain relationship than are any of the other techniques or metaphors previously discussed. It, too, is primarily a data extraction and classification technique that emphasizes the pattern of responses in a novel conceptual manner. Should the vectors created from the combination of pixel-level responses be sufficiently different from one cognitive process to another, they may help us to distinguish between cognitive states in the same sense that a biomarker may indicate some behavioral or function or, more likely, clinical dysfunction.

A further limitation to the application of MVPA is a practical one; despite their conceptual attractiveness, the most successful applications of MVPA techniques for cognitive neuroscience have been in the domain of visual perception where the neural responses maintain their topological relationships to the stimulus. The MVPA techniques have been applied most successfully in this context by Haynes and Rees (2005) and Kamitani and Tong (2005) to distinguish differential responses to line orientation, for example. Because line orientation is preserved at least topologically constant at the early levels of the visual system, an almost exact (if distorted) mapping of the stimulus pattern is possible. At higher cognitive levels, where the topology is not maintained and the neural representation may have a symbolic rather than an isomorphic relationship to the stimulus, even this powerful technique may be inapplicable. The few examples of higher level cognitive processes (Poldrack, Halchenko, & Hanson, 2009; Shinkareva et al., 2008), for example, that have been approached from this new vantage point are not compelling because studies of this kind are biased by sensory (i.e., isomorphic) properties of the system. As Poldrack and his colleagues (2009) noted:

> Substantial variability was present in sensory cortices; given the fact that the different studies [the cognitive tasks] varied substantially in the visual stimulus characteristics and the presence of auditory stimuli, this was not surprising, and it suggested that classification does not necessarily reflect the higher-order cognitive aspects of the task.
>
> *(p. 1366)*

Like all other forms of data analysis, the vectors or the MVPA decision spaces by means of which the neural findings are categorized are not, in any sense of the word, explanatory theories of mind-brain relations. MVPA programs are very useful methods for extracting, collecting, and organizing data. At their best, they can identify different vectors (i.e., patterns of responses) that can be associated with different cognitive processes. Nevertheless, they remain neutral with regard to specific neural states except in the most general way—for example, by emphasizing that brain responses to a stimulus or task are widely distributed rather than localized.

This point has been elaborated on by Klein (2011), who argues that "Significance tests alone cannot provide evidence of the functional structure of causally dense systems, including the brain." He goes on to say that, "Images are not evidence of how the brain works" (p. 265). They can only point us to regions where the salient activity resides—if they are actually localized in any particular region.

Thus, despite the fact that metaphors suggested by MVPA methods can act as heuristics and suggest new ways of thinking about the organization of this complex organ, they also remain neutral with regard to the exact mechanisms of psychoneural equivalence in the same way an average value tells us nothing about the original data or the accumulations and manipulations that produced that value. Indeed, within the limits defined by the many sources of variability influencing these techniques, no MVPA findings may be in conflict with any other; they just represent different ways of summarizing the data.

Nevertheless, the introduction of MVPA techniques is promising; even if not capable of completely solving the mind-brain problem, it may change the way we conceptualize brain activity by both reducing the scale of our metaphors and releasing us from the conceptual constraints of locale-specific encoding.

4.6   Challenges to MCT Theory Building

Having now discussed some specific examples of MCT-type theories, it is clear that there are a number of technical and conceptual challenges faced by those attempting to develop this kind of theory of cognition. In the following section, I consider some of the most obvious difficulties faced by MCT theoreticians operating at the macroneural level.

The Unified Stream of Consciousness: One of the main obstacles to building an MCT is the extreme difficulty of fitting the psychological phenomenology of a "Jamesian" unified stream of consciousness with the basic idea of a macroneural neural network that is made up of many separate components.[11] Any effort to break up such a unified cognitive process into a set of discrete subcomponents or modules corresponding to localized brain regions is obstructed by the arbitrariness of psychological taxonomies. Indeed, the whole idea of a network of separable parts or modules or nodes may reflect an incorrect predisposition to attempt to solve difficult problems by breaking them up into parts according to the "methode" championed by Descartes; an idea that may destroy the very global representation for which we seek. This traditional approach is also challenged by a more holistic view of both the mind and the brain—a new metaphor that now seems to be emerging from new empirical evidence.

At the microneuronal levels, we have neurons, entities whose discrete component nature cannot be denied. However, at the macroneural level, the brain is not quite so obviously made up of precisely defined discrete components. Despite Brodmann's use of the various architectonic fields of neuronal types, the macroneural areas that he identified are not clearly demarcated from each other either functionally or anatomically. Thus, dividing the whole brain into reliable and meaningful components or locales that can be matched, individually, or collectively, to cognitive processes may be an unproductive and misleading strategy. In addition, our attention may be further misdirected by the easy availability of methods and tools such as the fMRI that are designed to search for spatially localized activity. Thus, the possibility that we are responding much too strongly to both iconic preconceptions and available methodologies in our attempts to compartmentalize the brain cannot be ignored.

Stimuli Are Not the Immediate Causal Agent: Another challenge is to define the actual cognitive processes being compared with macroneural brain responses. In general, psychologists are not able to control the cognitive states that actually drive the brain responses simply by structuring the stimuli. Often ambiguous tasks such as "thinking" or "attention" generate confounding cognitive states over which we have limited control. Major differences in cognitive activity can arise because of interpretive differences on the part of a subject of the meaning of a stimulus or intentional efforts to "clear the mind," or even to play games with the experimenter. In short, what a stimulus is meant to mean by the experimenter is not always what it actually means to a subject. Of course, the hope is that as psychology gets better and better at defining its stimuli, that variability in the salient cognitive responses may become increasingly well controlled.

Noise: Just as we cannot control the actual cognitive response to an ambiguous stimulus, we cannot always eliminate spurious signals and background noise from the environment. For example, Langers and van Dijk (2011) attributed major differences in BOLD activations to the "ubiquitous influence of acoustic scanner noise on alertness and arousal" (p. 1617). This kind of noise affects not only the acoustic response but also vision, working memory, and most seriously for good control, the default response. In addition, there is considerable psychological and neurophysiological variability that has to be treated as uncontrolled noise.

Intractability: A major intellectual challenge for MCT development is the possibility that in searching for the solution to the mind-brain problem, we may have set out on what is an impossible quest. It is well known in mathematical circles that there are intractable problems that are much simpler than those posed by cognitively significant neural networks of nodes and tracts. For example, the physical three-body problem is not considered to be solvable in a general way.[12] If we cannot analyze the behavior of a simple group of three planetary bodies interacting under the influence of a single uniform force—gravity—then what is the basis of the overly optimistic expectation that we should be able to understand the operation of a cognitively significant macroneural neural network of even as few as a dozen or more idiosyncratically interacting nodes?

The Uncertainty of the Existence of Nodes: A further problem is that of simply determining that a node actually exists and that it is functionally relevant. In most brain imaging studies, for example, a node is a probabilistic entity—that is, its existence is dependent on statistical tests and is, therefore, fraught with the possibility of false alarms and misses. Decisions about the presence or absence of a node may depend on the arbitrariness of an experimenter's predilection to set the imaging threshold relatively high or relatively low. Nodes, therefore, may slip into and out of existence on the basis of arbitrary criterion.

In this vein, there is a further suggestion emerging from recent research that a *functional* "node" may not correspond to a discrete and stable *anatomical* region of the brain. Wang et al. (2010) proposed an extraordinary idea that may change our views of what we mean by a node and by terms such as localization or distribution. The traditional view, enhanced by the fMRI technology, is that a node is geographically or anatomically located at a particular place on the brain. The MCT theories discussed in this book implicitly make this assumption. One implication of Wang et al.'s work, however, is that, for the resting state at least, anatomically and stable localized nodes do not exist; instead, a node may consist of a transitory array of salient responsive regions distributed over broad regions of the brain. The appearance of a geographically isolated "node" may have to be replaced by the *functional synchrony* rather than their *geographical proximity*. This would seriously complicate our attempts to develop an MCT based on the kind of spatial data obtainable from brain imaging devices simply because these regions may not permanently exist.

Modularization: Indeed, the problem of whether the brain (as well as the mind) can be modularized has become a matter of concern in recent years. Since the matter was first raised by Fodor (1983), there has been an ongoing debate about the existence of cognitive modules. The question, then, naturally arises for cognitive neuroscience: Are modules merely a convenient way of parsing and organizing a complex problem, or are they a realistic expression of the functional anatomy of the brain and the modules of the mind? Arguments appear on both sides (see, for example, the discussions by Friston & Price, 2011; Henson, 2011; and Sternberg, 2011). Much of their discussion has been framed in formal mathematical terms. I believe, to the contrary, that the question is primarily an empirical one for the brain and an arguable and an arbitrary one for cognition. Indeed, as we see later, recent evidence suggests that brain modules (i.e., specialized activation areas) do not exist; rather the brain seems to acting more as a whole than as a collection of interacting macroscopic parts.

Functional Specificity: An additional challenge to MCT development is that many MCT models depend upon the idea that the putative "nodes" are function-specific. Thus, MCT theories imply that a node is responsible for or associated with a particular cognitive process. However, an abundance of research now suggests that no brain region is associated exclusively and permanently with any particular cognitive process; instead, each is better considered as a temporary constituent part of a system whose function may vary from one cognitive state to the next.

Regions of Interest: Furthermore, the use of preliminary estimates of where a node is located (for example, when one is defining "functional region of interest") may be necessary to constrain the brain regions that must be studied in a complex experiment. However, such a procedure may also bias the outcome of an otherwise well-designed experiment as noted by Friston, Rotshtein, Geng, Sterzer, & Henson (2006).

Underdetermination: In addition, from the outset of any effort to develop an overarching MCT theory, there is the continuing problem of underdetermination. That is, even if highly correlated and significant, the observations that we make about cognitive processes and neural networks are insufficient to distinguish between the many possible explanatory networks that could implement a plausible solution to the problem. Given that there may be no unique solution—individuals may have dissimilar neural strategies depending on their previous experience—the task at hand may be impossible.

Other Challenges: Ramsey et al. (2010) also provided an insightful list of some of the analytical problems facing the mind-brain theoretician after the data collection phase has been completed. In brief paraphrase, their list includes the following:

1. Selecting the best possible theory from among the large number of possible theories
2. Accounting for indirect influences of cryptic nonlinear effects that are not directly measured
3. Accounting for and modeling individual differences
4. Handling overlapping but different putative networks
5. Resolving conduction time uncertainties
6. Sequential dependencies among responses

Important caveats concerning the role of the theoretical tools that are available to study the mind-brain relationship remain; despite mathematical power and experimental design ingenuity, the task of relating cognitive and neural processes remains extremely difficult. A major reason is that the intrinsic variability and combinatorial complexity of the neural representations of the responses to the cognitive tasks may deny us robust empirical correlations.

Another reason is that we may be barking up the wrong tree in a very fundamental way—the macroneural level at which much current research is being carried out may not be the one at which the necessary and sufficient information processes producing cognitive experience are occurring. Thus, we may be seeking a nonexistent chimera or a partially random process that may never produce the robust, deterministic theories to which we aspire. Similarly, the search for a unique explanation of how brain activity is transformed into cognitive activity may fall victim to the differences between the varying cognitive strategies used by different individuals.

In an interesting and very relevant article, Smith et al. (2011), while describing a number of methods that may be used to model and analyze networks, also list many of the potential artifacts that could bias the outcome of a neural network calculation. Their comments are generally relevant to the challenges facing MCT development. The overarching problem, already mentioned, is that there are organizational properties of networks that can individually or collectively make a simple problem into an intractable one. The potential sources of difficulty for network theories identified by Smith et al. include the following:

1. A common time series acting over the whole network
2. Multiple inputs
3. Multiple outputs due to inaccurate estimates of nodes
4. Feedback connections between nodes
5. Cyclic connections between nodes
6. Multiple connections between nodes
7. Strength of connections
8. Connection strength changes
9. Time-varying connections
10. Temporal smoothing due to haemodynamic smoothing

An additional problem in evaluating the validity of any proposed MCT is that the connections between nodes implied by the sequential activations of the multitude of regional responses are not necessarily the same as the ones determined by other criteria such as anatomical dissection, dye infusion, or Diffusion Tensor Imaging (DTI) methods. A distinction made by Friston (1994) between structural, functional, and effective connectivity, therefore, becomes especially germane in this context. By structural connectivity, Friston was referring to the physical pathways that can be demonstrated with anatomical methods as simple as a scalpel, as complicated as a DTI, or by retrograde injection of tracer chemicals. Because of the allusion to structure or anatomy, there is tendency for us to refer to these as the "real" connections. However, none of the observed structural connections by themselves can tell us anything about the main question of interest to cognitive psychologists—how does all of this circuitry encode the mind?

Furthermore, Friston's concept of "functional connectivity" depends on measurements made with fMRI techniques in response to cognitive stimuli or tasks. On the basis of various criteria, interactions between putative nodes are suggested by functional relations; for example, by concomitant or sequential activations, cross correlations with and without delays, and other statistical, both temporal and spatial, interdependencies. Such evidence can also highlight functional relationships between neural nodes along tracts that are not known anatomically. In this case the determination of connectivity is indirect; connections are made on the basis of inferences, often of a statistical nature, drawn from the locations and sequences in which various parts of the brain become activated.

Effective connectivity, according to Friston, adds the concept of directionality and, thus, is a more likely statement of causal influences when added to the implied functional connections. However, effective connectivity is always suspect because bidirectional links and multiple interconnections with lateral, feed forward, and feedback can make it difficult to determine where an activation is initiated, much less its role in a complex network; in other words, there is great uncertainty about the hierarchy—the order of activation—of the nodes in a system.

Another problem raised by Friston is that there may be disagreement between anatomical, on the one hand, and effective or functional connectivity, on the other. That is, the system may be of such a high level of complexity that what appear to functional connections may not coincide with the observed structural ones. In some basic sense, of course, this cannot be true; functions cannot be carried out in a disembodied form without some structure. To suggest otherwise is to slip into dualist thinking that has no place in cognitive neuroscience. Beyond that ontological caveat, any discrepancy between anatomically identifiable and functional or effective connections raises serious questions about the meaning of each of the latter two types.

In all of the preceding discussion of particular theories, therefore, it is best to keep in mind that the structural and functional networks must eventually coincide. If not, then rethinking of the whole idea of determining the interconnections, as well as the resulting theories, must be reconsidered. It is not at all certain that our methods are powerful enough to guarantee that function can be the measure of specific structure. It is also clear that the dynamic nature of the brain could strongly affect our views of functional connectivity models whereas we should expect the structural networks to remain stable barring surgical intervention or trauma.

4.7   Interim Summary

The most perplexing question is whether MCT-type theories, the current state of the theoretical art, are the best that can be done in the context of cognitive neuroscience? Are we at an impasse beyond which we cannot proceed? Or, to the contrary, are we momentarily just at the foot of a surmountable barrier, constrained by inadequate methods, particularly computational power and MRI systems resolution? It is impossible to definitively resolve futurist questions of this kind—surprising breakthroughs are inevitable; however, given the complexity of the problem and the "in principle" barriers to analysis that constrain us currently, it may be that the macroneural approach is fundamentally limited as an entrée into understanding the great mind-brain conundrum.

The most pessimistic answer to the question of future prospects of MCT is driven by the potential failure of macroneural connectionist concepts of "nodes" and "tracts"—the foundations of so many current theoretical contributions. It can be argued in light of new research that the widely held concept of mental processes emerging from the activity of networks of localized macroneural brain activation sites is simply misguided—it is the wrong level of analysis at which to find cognition. However, the problems plaguing this approach to the mind-brain problem are immense and must eventually become better known to cognitive neuroscientists, some of whom currently tread along the fringes of posing intractable problems.

This difficulty aside, there is an even more devastating possibility looming on the horizon of all network theories based on the existence of "nodes" or demarcatable activation regions. That question concerns the actual reality of the nodes: Are they real neurophysiological responses or are they statistical artifacts?

Critical evaluations of the entire MCT approach are the topic of the next chapter.

Notes

1. As we see in Chapter 5, an emerging problem is that "many" cognitive neuroscience experiments using fMRI protocols do not report their procedures in adequate enough detail to permit clear-cut replications (Carp, 2012a). The question thus arises, what does this literature mean if a large proportion of it cannot be replicated? The question might also be asked, is this lack of replication psychobiologically inherent or just a manifestation of modern technology?

2. I use the word "ontology" more in the traditional philosophical sense. An ontology in philosophy is a statement about the nature of reality often unaccompanied by any empirical evidence; it may be based on assumptions and conjectures that have arisen from inductive interpretations. Thus, my meaning comes closer to the a priori postulates or axioms of an initial point of view than it does to the ex post facto concept of Price and Friston. Poldrack, on the other hand, seems to use the term more in the sense that I use "taxonomy"—as an organized body of knowledge. The more serious remaining question is, do these proposed "ontologies" accurately model the psychobiological system of interest?

3. Of course, Mesulam also based his work on a long tradition of research in physiological psychology that unequivocally demonstrated the interaction of the various parts of the brain when surgically lesioned or electrically stimulated or simply dissected.

4. It should also be reiterated that not all "neural network" models are actually neural in the sense I use it here. A number of authors have developed theories that are networks based on the function of cognitive processes without making any connection to the specific neurophysiology or neuroanatomy of the system. For example, Houghton, Tipper, Weaver, and Shore (1996) developed a compelling mathematical model of selective attention that describes the hypothetical function of such a system. Indeed, it is also a network model, as evidenced in their figures and discussion. However, it was done independently of any neurophysiological data or theories specifying the role of particular neural elements; it was based exclusively on behavioral data. This is what I have referred to as a descriptive theory. It is not a neuroreductive theory in the sense I use the word here. Simply introducing neural vocabulary adds little meaning to what otherwise might be considered to be "functional descriptions."

5. A logistic regression is a means of predicting the probability of binary (i.e., yes-no) responses. In this case, it refers to the probability that a particular brain region would be activated or deactivated in a particular cognitive task.

6. Baddeley's (Baddeley & Hitch, 1974) psychological theory of working memory is considered by many to have been one of the most informative influences on modern theories of working memory. It is based on the idea of multiple components, each of

which has some particular function. As such, it stimulated the idea that there are multiple corresponding brain areas for each cognitive component and each brain region may have multiple functions. As a result, we no longer take localized function-specificity as a sine qua non of MCT theories.

7. In an earlier book (Uttal, 2012, Figure 3.7) and in the summary of Chapter 5 of this book, I compared the results of an array of meta-analytic studies in which the supposed neural components of working memory were described. Each of these studies was essentially a qualitative prototheory of which macroneural cortical regions were involved in working memory. I concluded that there was still no agreement even among the data-rich meta-analyses and that the observed inconsistency between these analyses did not yet support an acceptable neuroreductive theory of this very important cognitive process. The example of the work of Schroll et al. (2012) that I use here is distinguished more by its mathematical tests than by its claim that it resolves this inconsistency.

8. An interesting side point, given the fact that this is a recent macroneural theory of cognition, is that very few of the neurophysiological justifications are based on any brain imaging data. A search for "fMRI" in their article turned up only one use of the word in their references.

9. In a personal communication with Schroll, I was advised that they used the word "neuron" (and, presumably, neuronal properties such as membrane potentials and firing rates) "in a rather abstract way (a more neutral term could be 'unit') . . . we did not model neuronal spikes (action potentials)." (H. Schroll, personal communication, March 2, 2012). From my point of view, because all of the supporting empirical evidence was macroneural, it would have been preferable to deal with the outputs of the model in completely macroneural terms rather than to suddenly leap to a microneuronal vocabulary of neuronal response rates, as they did.

10. Any of my readers interested in pursuing some of the details of multidimensional pattern analysis will find detailed discussions in Haxby (2010) and in Norman, Polyn, Detre, and Haxby (2006).

11. Although this is referred to as one version of the binding problem, it is unlikely that binding is other than a pseudoproblem. To the extent that the overall state of a network can be considered to be the psychoneural equivalent of mental activity, there is no obvious need to seek some means of reconstructing parts that were torn asunder only for reasons of conceptual or experimental convenience. For an extended discussion of the binding problem, see the article by M. Vacariu and G. Vacariu (2010).

12. The three-body problem in classical physics is tasked with determining the subsequent trajectories of three objects that are under the mutual influence of a single kind of force (i.e., gravity) from their initial conditions of mass, position, and velocity. In general, it is considered to be unsolvable unless constrained by making one of the bodies very small or very distant from the other two. However, approximate solutions are possible in special cases. Clearly, however, the technical difficulty of studying the interaction of a multitude of neurons under the influence of idiosyncratic synaptic interconnections is far more difficult. For example, several decades ago Leon D. Harmon demonstrated that a set of only three simulated neurons (neuromimes in his vocabulary) produced unpredictable patterns of activity.

5

ADDITIONAL CRITIQUES OF MACRONEURAL CONNECTIONIST THEORIES

5.1 The Thesis

In this chapter, I further challenge the locationist prototheory or metaphor that currently dominates thinking in cognitive neuroscience by reviewing additional critiques that have been made in the last few years. I argue that these critiques are now becoming insistent as part of the argument that much of the macroneural approach epitomized by fMRI findings and theories must be considered to be a flawed enterprise in which statistical anomalies, a variety of sources of bias, and conflated predilections often replace reliable data as the most influential but erroneous forces in our theory construction. I further argue that however good we may be in extracting, tabulating, and organizing data,[1] major portions of this theoretical corpus contribute little to explaining how cognitive processes actually emerge from neural activity. Nor is there anything that points to any potential resolution of this situation in the foreseeable future. In short, the thesis presented here contends that correlations between macroneural and cognitive processes are misreadings of what are essentially stochastic processes[2] that, as a result of their partially random properties, have little to do with understanding the neural basis of cognitive processes once we probe beyond the sensory and motor transmission codes.

My arguments are based on logical and empirical postulates and data that limit the basic validity and reliability of current findings. There is nothing supernatural or inexplicable in principle about this state of affairs; all involved in modern cognitive neuroscience agree that the brain is in some way the basis of cognitive processes and that, whatever the underlying processes are, they are extraordinarily complex and the salient level of components too numerous to process. There is so much to discover about both the brain and cognition that few investigators have applied the most powerful litmus test for good science—public replicability. Unfortunately, because of the rich lode of possible experimental variables, few experiments in cognitive neuroscience are conscientiously replicated and, in the few instances in which they are, earlier results have all-too-often not been replicated.

Like any other science, powerful personal, social, practical, and economic forces, as well as the grand intellectual and scientific impulses toward understanding for its own part, drive today's cognitive neuroscience's empirical and theoretical activities. Individual gain and notoriety, available instrumentation and facilities, and inadequately substantiated assumptions based on the prevailing Zeitgeist all contribute to misreading or misinterpreting available findings.

How could this misdirection of a significant portion of the efforts of so large a scientific community have occurred? Some insight into a possible answer to this question can be obtained by considering the flow of ideas from cognitive neuroscience axioms and postulates to derived theory and practice. What scientists think and do is strongly influenced by their basic postulates; in cognitive neuroscience, in particular, incorrect basic postulates produce effects that can propagate down through the entire scientific corpus of knowledge—classic as well as current. The influence of basic postulates is exacerbated today by the sheer power of modern technology to measure and analyze signals that were completely inaccessible only a few decades ago. In fact, what these powerful machines are able to do now forces certain perspectives on us. Thus, a machine that measures localized brain activities (e.g., an fMRI) imposes the basic concept of spatial localization on our entire scientific system. Similarly, a system that measures temporal excursions (e.g., an EEG) impels us toward a perspective on brain activities based on time and temporal variables. It is not always the case, however, that these perspectives are congruent with the actual organization of the brain; nevertheless, the complexity of the mind-brain problem offers many opportunities for us to detect what seem to be the sought for kinds of organization in our findings—whether or not they actually exist.

Another purpose of this chapter is to present the case for the proposition that no complete macroneural theory of the mind-brain yet exists or is likely to exist in the foreseeable future—only vague metaphors of how the brain might be organized appear on the distant horizon. One leg of this argument is the very basic empirical fact that brain images may very well be artifacts—weakly correlated signals of cognitive activity rather than the hoped for "holy grail" of macroneural neuroreductionism. As we see, there is also suggestive new evidence that when subject samples sizes are sufficiently large and the statistical methods do not prejudge a particular outcome, the postulate of localized activation regions or nodes as tangible entities disappears.

A second leg of this argument is that the data obtained with fMRI systems are unacceptably unreliable and inconsistent. Therefore, it is difficult for these macroneural measures to provide the basis for a robust theory of mind-brain relations. At the very least in any science, one must have confidence in the data and observations on which a theory is ultimately to be based. If the data are not strong, then all of the theorizing in the world cannot make a "silk purse" of it.

My goals here are to point out, first, that there are both empirical and conceptual problems with the entire enterprise in which macroneural brain images are associated with cognitive processes; second, to identify the causes for this problem; and, third, to argue that macroneural brain images are not even well enough correlated with cognitive processes to justify their role in the formulation of plausible prototheories of mind-brain relations. To do this, I also examine some of the critiques and countercritiques that have arisen in recent years.

5.2   Factors Influencing Theory Development

In the main, theories in psychology (especially those that link cognitive and neural data) tend to die off rather than to be disproved, remaining only as vestiges, as new ideas come into play. As brain-relevant science matured, traditional ideas such as extreme cortical localization have diminished in both application and theoretical importance. The main reason for their demise usually was simply changes in relevant empirical evidence. When a science confronts inconsistent data and results or when the implications of fallacious theories become evident, earlier approaches simply tend to fade away.[3] As the importance of reliable empirical evidence should be the standard of the scientific approach, those fields that could not withstand this kind of scrutiny should rapidly diminish in relevance although still leaving their footprints in our theories.

New methodological approaches to science also contribute to the rejection or, hopefully, to the evolution of some of the older protosciences. The engineering development of new instruments in recent years opened the doors to new kinds of experiments, to sometimes astonishing new findings and data and, ultimately, to new ideas. New experimental protocols, as opposed to failures in logic and speculation, emerge as the most effective means of burying what so often turn out to be pseudosciences. In particular, the application of statistical methods (including the simple but powerful concept of control groups) led to our modern empirical approach to studying every science in which variability was an issue; none more needy than the cognitive neurosciences. Just as the limitations and properties of these older protosciences were eventually contradicted by the very empirical data they invoked for support, so, too, are current macroneural findings beginning to suggest that the prototheories they stimulated may be due for some major changes, if not outright replacement by new metaphors.

5.3   Macroneural Theories of Mind—The Current Situation

The financial and intellectual investment in cognitively related brain imaging research in the last 20 years has been extraordinary in the history of cognitive neuroscience. It expanded research from a "small science" culture in which individual investigators, perhaps with a few students and very limited budgets, probed, stimulated, recorded from, or surgically lesioned the brain into "big science" projects in which large teams of investigators with a variety of skills and training gathered around multimillion dollar facilities.

The ultimate goal of this new wave of cognitive "big science" research, like that of its predecessors, was to help us toward understanding how the brain produces mental functions. The promise that balanced out the high costs of this new approach was that signals from the brain might be indicators or, even better, the mechanisms (i.e., the psychoneural equivalents) of cognitive process. The simple fact that the signals were coming from the brain gave them compelling face validity. Ideally, macroneural brain images constituted information-bearing indicators of what the brain was doing during cognitive activity. On the other hand, the fact that many early studies of brain responses only weakly and inconsistently correlated with cognitive activity was an unappreciated harbinger of things to come.

The initial and prevailing initial postulate during the first decade of brain imaging research was that the brain was organized in the manner that had been originally suggested by the phrenologists; that is, it was composed of a collection of function-specific and uniquely localized regions of the brain. Indeed, early on there was a flood of research reports that actually connected specific regions of the brain with particular cognitive activities.

In the second decade of brain imaging research, quite a different consensus gradually emerged under the pressure of new empirical facts. That emerging perspective was that single (or a few) isolated regions could not possibly represent cognitive processes because many regions of the brain were being activated by any cognitive task. Therefore, the idea of a system of multiple interconnected brain components or localized nodes emerged. As I have already discussed in earlier chapters, this was a profoundly different concept from the neophrenological theories of the first decade that had led to the still-persisting idea that highly specific individual cognitive modules were encoded by localized, function-specific locations.

The idea of multiple sites as the representational mechanisms of cognitive processes was a fundamental change in thinking about brain organization; it was epitomized by the idea of a system of interconnected activation sites (or, as they came to be called, "nodes") as opposed to the initial notion of isolated, unique function-specific activation regions. These interconnected systems, idealized as MCT theories, were, it was proposed, the true correlates of cognitive processes. Virtually all research was by the turn of the 21st century producing results that showed multiple activation regions; it is on this basis that most macroneural connectionist prototheories of brain action were subsequently constructed. Analytic methods of this kind are often formulated as graph theoretical structures that depended on the preliminary identification of the nodes, some idea of at least the functional interconnections between the nodes and, most important of all, their relation to cognitive processes.

Network prototheories are, however, only a step towards the emerging concept of a fully distributed cognitive nervous system. No longer are specific psychological functions attributed to unique and isolated activation areas. Instead, many, if not all, parts of the brain are currently thought to be simultaneously involved in the representation of a cognitive process. However, the localization postulate is still very much a part of this theoretical approach—the individual nodes having morphed into multiple nodes that themselves are presumed to be narrowly localized and function-specific.

5.4   Critiques and Countercritiques

Increasingly, however, evidence is accruing (e.g., Barrett & Satpute, 2013; Oosterwijk et al., 2012) that very broadly, if not universally, distributed regions of the brain are nonspecifically activated during cognitive processing. It is the relation among widely separated portions of the brain that may actually reflect the macroneural activity of the underlying microneuronal networks, but probably in a transitory and highly variable manner. According to investigators like these and others to be introduced shortly, there are no specific places in the brain that account for a particular cognitive process; instead, most of the brain seems to be involved in a wide variety of cognitive processes in a nonspecific manner. Oosterwijk et al. (2012) also argued against function-specific and localized cognitive modules or faculties as well. In their words:

> Growing evidence points to the hypothesis that diverse mental states emerge from the combination of domain-general psychological processes or "ingredients" that map to large scale distributed networks in association regions of the brain.
>
> *(p. 2110)*

It is problematical how many of the goals and expectations concerning the promise of the brain imaging methodology have been realized. It seems that a cottage industry has grown up in which the conceptual and empirical bases of brain imaging has been challenged. A few clear voices have arisen out of the cacophony of both supportive and critical voices that clarify what the problem issues are. Among the most notable of these edifying and clarifying contributions is the work of Farah (2014). In a remarkably well-balanced and fair article, she identifies many of the counterarguments against the brain imaging approach as she "critiques [the] critiques" (p. S19). Farah is no ideologue; she stakes out a middle position in the following manner.

> In the spirit of healthy skepticism, I will critically examine these criticisms themselves. Each contains at least a kernel of truth, although I will argue that in some cases the kernel has been overextended in ways that are

inaccurate or misleading. In other cases, the criticism are valid as presented and deserve the careful attention of imaging researchers.

(p. S19)

Farah's clarification and identification of the bases of current criticisms of brain imaging as a tool for cognitive psychology sums up each criticism, suggests what its "intended scope" is intended to be, and provides a nutshell evaluation of each particular criticism. The following list abstracts and paraphrases Farah's counterarguments (or agreements) with each of the criticisms she identifies:

1. **Blood Not Brain:** Yes, functional brain images are indirect measures, but so, too, are many other measures in sciences that have been productive in theory building. There is a causal relationship between blood measures and brain activity although we do not know it—yet.
2. **Fabrications:** Yes, color codes are arbitrary, uncalibrated, and potentially deceptive. However, this is a problem for all kinds of data displays.
3. **Localization:** Yes, Farah agrees, localization is a "questionable goal," but most research these days is aimed at other problems removed from localization per se. She argues that much of today's work is being done on adaptation paradigms, the state of the entire brain, functional connectivity, and multidimensional pattern analysis.
4. **Cannot Test Psychological Theories:** Although, according to some investigators, no theory has ever been confirmed by a brain image (Coltheart, 2006), Farah argues this is true of virtually all psychological research because of the underdetermination problems (i.e., we do not have access to unique distinctions between theories). However, she sees some yet unrealized hope in establishing such discriminations by brain imaging techniques.
5. **Brain Images Bias Hypotheses:** Brain imaging (as a major tenet of this present book professes), like the measurements obtained with any other kind of instrumentation, does drive hypotheses. Brain images support modularization, but there are other methods going on in parallel that would contradict this bias. Concurrent methods will lead to converging evidence that justifies hypotheses generated by brain imaging techniques.
6. **"Wanton Reverse Inference":** Farah agrees with Poldrack's (2006) very important admonition against any effort to identify an ongoing cognitive process from a brain image (reverse inference) except in some extraordinary circumstances—despite the fact that forward inference (determining the neural response to a cognitive stimulus or state) can be done in principle.
7. **"Slippery Statistics":** Because of the variability and such other factors as poor signal-to-noise ratios of brain activity, they, like all other

sciences, must be processed by statistical methods. This can lead to false or misleading responses and then to incorrect hypotheses. Farah accepts that these problems are real but endemic in modern science. She argues that reality may vary with statistical method and urges care in evaluating images.

8. **Influence:** Finally, Farah points out that brain images may be too "convincing" or "appealing." She suggests that they exert an inordinate amount of influence on hypothesis generation or theory building. Again she concludes that this is "not unique to neuroscience."

Farah performed a useful service in crystallizing the criticisms against functional brain imaging in its current states. In general she concludes the following:

> Each of these criticisms contains an element of truth but overextends that element to mistakenly cast doubt on the validity or utility of functional neuroimaging research as a whole. None of the criticism reviewed here constitute reasons to reject or even drastically curtail the use of neuroimaging. Rather they remind us that neuroimaging, like other scientific methods, is subject to various specific errors that the self-correcting process continues to address.
>
> *(p. S28)*

Farah's presentation is so balanced and even-handed that it is difficult to take issue with any of the countercriticisms she raises. However, in reading and rereading her comments, one must appreciate that there are several incompletenesses in it that should not be overlooked in any reasoned argument about the utility of macroneural signals in producing a valid theory. First, is her repeated suggestion that many of the criticisms of brain imaging are typical of any science (e.g., theories are often built on indirect evidence). This type of counterargument ignores the special problems that are generated when research attempts to cross boundaries between objective (tangible) and subjective (inaccessible) measures—the hallmark of cognitive neuroscience. The mind-brain problem is not just another scientific problem, but one that lies at the apex of complexity and combinatoric plausibility. There is probably no more challenging issue confronting science than the gap between the intangible mind and the tangible brain. Although cognition-brain theory shares many constraints with other sciences, it also has, by virtue of its goals, special susceptibility to some of them.

It is difficult to counter arguments that are based on such "soft" criteria as hope and expectation in the absence of robust empirical evidence. Yet many of Farah's counterarguments seem to be based on just these factors or idealizations of the anticipated role of science in explaining our world. There are well-known limits in science that preclude certain kinds of progress. Consider for example the role of the second law of thermodynamics on the possibility of perpetual motion machines or the Lorentz transformations on the speed of light. These are limits in physics, and some of us argue that equivalent limits exist in cognitive neuroscience.

A further observation is that Farah's list of criticisms and countercriticisms of brain imaging is very incomplete and new challenges are raised virtually every day.

The following list briefly summarizes some of the other critiques not identified by Farah but raised by one or another skeptic of fMRI-cognitive research.

1. **Complexity:** The number of neurons and interconnections is so great that modern combinatorial mathematics rejects any possibility of a computational solution to the mind-brain problem.
2. **Level of Analysis:** The macroneural level at which brain imaging measurements are being made is not the microneuronal level at which material brain become intangible cognition.
3. **Loss of Information:** Because of the statistical nature of most brain imaging methodology, almost all germane microneuronal information is lost. Data pooled are data lost.
4. **Underdetermination:** There is insufficient information in brain imaging data to develop an explanatory theory.
5. **Inaccessibility:** Because a person's thoughts and mental experiences are arguably private and inaccessible to measurement (through either experiment or introspection), there is no solid anchor against which to compare brain images. Furthermore, experimentation is directed at a moving target because our mental activities are constantly changing.
6. **Replication Is Rare:** Because of inadequate reporting, it is rare to find brain imaging findings being replicated (Carp, 2012a).
7. **Multiple Analytic Pathways:** Because of the multiple ways that data can be analyzed, interpretations are equivocal (Carp, 2012b).
8. **Sensory and Motor Transmission Coding Is Not Cognitive Coding:** Although we have had great success in decoding transmission codes, for many reasons this success is not an indicator that equally compelling success is just over the horizon.
9. **Vague Definitions of Key Terminologies and Anatomical Structures:** The cognitive vocabulary used in cognitive neuroscience is vague and imprecise. It is never quite clear whether two experiments are studying the same or different phenomena.
10. **Additional Statistical Criticisms:** Farah only scratches the surface of the statistical problems facing cognitive brain imaging typified by a continued stream of misunderstandings, misuses, and misinterpretations of basic and not-so-basic statistics. Although quite properly highlighting the work on multiple comparisons and circularity, her examples do not convey the full range of errors in statistical analysis now becoming

evident. Not the least of these is ignoring Yule's (1926) famous admonition *not to mistake correlation for causation.*

11. **Natural Variability:** Natural variability in brain size, shape, and locations add uncertainty to any reported localization.

12. **Inadequate Power:** In this context, the power of most brain imaging experiments is low due to the high costs of running an adequate sample of subjects. Only recently have large databases been accumulating that can overcome this criticism, and most laboratories still are limited to only a few subjects for what are complicated and multivariate protocols. Indeed, in those few instances in which very large databases are used (e.g., Gonzalez-Castillo et al., 2012 and Thyreau et al., 2012) the more typical result is the involvement of the whole brain.

13. **Data Replicability:** Farah overlooks the most important component of the scientific enterprise: The quality of the empirical data. There is a continued question of the replicability of much of brain imaging data, even in situations in which intrasubject comparisons are being made. This should not be surprising given the highly adaptive capabilities of the brain, but it does make for less than robust empirical support for the prospect of developing brain image-based theories in particular.

There is a pervasive question revolving around the revolution in technique represented by brain imaging technology. Do the inferred modular components of a cognitive process (as defined by experimental psychologists) necessarily map in some repeatable and coherent way onto localized regions of the brain (as defined by neuroanatomists and neurophysiologists)? As widely accepted as this hypothesis is, there have been persistent logical reasons and now an increasing number of empirical reasons to question it. The psychological processes and phenomena for which localized representations are assumed may not necessarily be dimensionally isomorphic with the brain's natural spatial layout. The cognitive processes are, it must also be remembered, themselves typically the instantiation of our experimental designs and not necessarily of any simple property of functional behavior. Whether they are divisible into the "hypothetical constructs" or intervening "modules or faculties" that correspond to specific anatomical regions or structures of the brain is uncertain. If they are not "natural categories" into which cognitive processes can be parsed, why should we take them seriously as definers of brain regions?

The implications and inferences of hypotheses and theories must be empirically tested to determine if they continue to hold more generally as indicators of brain structure. However easy to put this essential step of the investigative process into words, it is typically not that simple. Indeed, it is conversely true that when you are dealing with systems whose stimuli are at least multifactorial and for which the actual triggering stimuli are obscure, whose responses are multidimensional and redundant, and for which there may be no direct relation of stimulus to cognitive response, the probability of finding any kind of a response that satisfies a priori theoretical judgments becomes greatly enhanced. There are simply too many possible biasing variables, many of which are not controlled, to have much confidence in macroneural experiments.

In sum, although extremely popular as a means of studying macroneural brain-cognitive relations, there is much to be learned about what fMRI-based brain images actually mean. It is yet to be determined whether they are doorways to understanding or are misleading us about the basic nature of the complex relationship between cognition and brain activities.

5.5   On Validity and Reliability

Two important questions now arise concerning macroneural levels of analysis and the theories and prototheories they generate. The first is whether the activation regions, peaks, or nodes are real. That is, are activation peaks valid correlates or indicators of localized cognitive activity or, to the contrary, are they merely artifacts of our expectations, misleading statistics, or technical artifacts that are unrelated to cognitive activity? The second question raises the issue of their reliability: Can results be replicated from one experiment or analysis to another?

There are many arguments, some of which I have discussed earlier and some newly considered here, that limit the contribution of fMRI findings to mind-brain theory. It may be fairly argued, for example, that the macroneural level of analysis with its spatial maps of brain activation is simply the wrong level of analysis at which to look for neural correlates of the mind. The BOLD signals from the brain may be the outcome of processes unrelated to cognitive functions rather than driven, correlated, or caused by those functions. For example, they might be analogues of the resonant response to the "impulse" represented by the onset of the stimulus in the manner that a bell will be stimulated to produce its characteristic ring when struck. In this context, the macroneural BOLD signal may have lost the critical microneuronal information during the successive stages of summation and accumulation that occur between the microneuronal network states and the macroneural brain image.

In the following sections of this chapter, I provide plausible empirical answers to the two important questions concerning validity and reliability, respectively:

1.   Are brain images valid indicators of cognitive activity? Specifically, do localized nodes actually exist?
2.   Are brain image data reliable?

On Validity: Are Localized Nodes Real?

The idea that brain image responses are localized regions of activity associable with cognitive processes has been central to the interpretation of brain images since the first application of functional imaging methods. For many years, the criterion for localizing a cognitive process in the brain has been the highest amplitude of the generated contrast. Cognition was assigned to a responding brain region because it was there that maximum differential activity was observed in control and experimental conditions. However, the actual magnitude and extent of a peak was always questionable because the response was determined not solely by the biology of the brain but also by the arbitrary nature of the threshold and significance criteria set by the investigator in designing his or her experimental protocols.

There has been a persistent and influential bias implicit in the theoretical approach taken by researchers since the beginning of cognitive neuroscience. That bias is the proclivity to concentrate on the discontinuous spatial properties of the brain; that is, on localized and spatially demarcated nodes. The brain has been mapped for years by spatial systems such as the Brodmann areas or the Talairach and Tournoux systems. Historically, the idea of specialized and separable locales on the brain has been the dominant metaphor of brain organization since the heyday of phrenology.

As a result of these factors and the limits or unsuitability of other technological approaches (e.g., single cell microelectrode methods and microneuronal networks of neurons) to the study of mind-brain relationships, cognitive neuroscientists have exhibited a predisposition to think about the brain primarily in terms of its macroneural spatial properties. The synergy between expectations and existing technology impelled students of cognitively related brain functions to traditionally seek spatial differences between experimental and control conditions. Nothing could be more natural in this context than to look for peaks of activity evoked by cognitive stimuli as the main macroneural clue to the brain's representational mechanisms underlying cognition. The metaphor of a sparse distribution of spatially extended nodes of activity fit well with the function-specific, localized model that dominated thinking about brain organization throughout the pre-fMRI days. Simple difference or subtractive measures of responses to experimental and control conditions were aimed early on to identify localized "peaks" of activity. The subtraction method has been criticized for many different reasons (e.g., Van Orden & Paap, 1997). The main problem with it, however, is that the macroneural measures are cumulative composites of the activity of a myriad of individual neurons. As such, the properties of the macroneural fMRI image are indeterminate with regard to what the network of underlying neurons may be doing. Exactly the same brain image may be produced by very different microneuronal network states. Thus, observations of "no difference" between fMRI responses may hide vast differences in the underlying neuronal network state.

Such approaches were also superficially consistent with much of the data reported over the last few decades; data accumulated that seemed to be supporting the idea of "hot spots," "localized responses," "nodes," or "activation peaks." The result, therefore, was that both logical and empirical pressures encouraged researchers to concentrate on data suggesting that there were discrete regions of activity, some of which were assumed to be closely related to cognitive processes.

The primary question concerning the validity of a more or less localized activation area can be expressed as follows: Do localized activation peaks isolatable from the rest of the brain's activity and putatively associated with cognitive processes, singly or in concert with others, actually exist? Because much of the research of the last two decades has been aimed at finding these activation peaks, a negative answer to this question would challenge the most basic assumptions of this kind of cognitive neuroscience. Nevertheless, the prevailing assumption that statistically significant peaks of activity can be distinguished from the background activity and that these nodes represent the activity of the parts of the brain that are selectively active during particular cognitive processes is rarely examined.

There are other possible and plausible answers to this "existence question" other than the current consensus. One answer is that the nodes are merely statistical artifacts that emerge from the complexity of what is essentially a partially random pattern of activation across the brain. As we shortly see, false nodes can be produced if the sample size of subjects or the number of trials is too small, if criterion levels are too low, or if the statistical analysis begs the questions by being biased towards the identification of peaks of maximum activity as opposed to some other form of organization.

There are a number of rarely considered arguments that suggest that the observed isolated peaks of activity are simply not valid in the formal sense that we are measuring what we think we are measuring. First, the amplitude and distribution of the significant peaks are typically very variable. Slight differences in experimental protocol can lead to massive differences in the nature of the brain image responses. Peaks came and went depending on statistical manipulations including, most importantly, the size of the sample of subjects. When sufficiently large numbers of subjects were used and data plotted simply in terms of the locations of individual activation peaks, nodal responses can be observed over broad regions of the brain as was shown earlier in Figure 2.1. This figure displays the typical appearance of the raw data that is to be gathered together for a meta-analysis—the locations of activation peaks that were deemed to be "significant"—before any pooling or statistical selection of the most salient regions.[4]

Figure 2.1 displays something very different from the few, sparsely localized activation peaks typical of earlier work; it shows that the raw peaks responding to the cognitive stimulus we call emotion were scattered over virtually all of the brain prior to the meta-analysis. It is only when such data are pooled, averaged, or meta-analyzed that some regions were identified as being more densely activated than were others and thus of special statistical and theoretical significance.

However, a very different interpretation of these raw data plots is possible. Clusters may reflect the natural variability of statistical distributions to occasionally exhibit regions of dense responses. These clusters, according to this hypothesis, may actually be statistical artifacts that would disappear under some conditions such as when adequately large amounts of data are involved in the computations.

Recently a number of investigators have reported data supporting just this alternative hypothesis. Gonzalez-Castillo et al. (2012), for example, suggested that the localized and sparse activation peaks are actually artifacts of inadequate sample sizes and statistical analysis methods that presupposed sparse localization. The alternative they proposed was that the salient regions of brain encoding cognitive processes were not isolated peaks but actually involved vast regions (up to 95%) of the brain.

To make this point, Gonzalez-Castillo and his colleagues averaged 500 trials from each of three subjects[5] in a letter-number discrimination task. They demonstrated that isolated "significant" peaks disappeared when these large samples of trials were used. Instead, there was a broad, undifferentiated response evoked over broad regions of the brain. Their point was that the "peaks" were not valid measures of cognition but artifacts of inadequate sample size and anticipatory statistical tools.

To further test these results, Gonzalez-Castillo and his colleagues hypothesized that the distributed extent of the evoked brain nodes should vary with the number of trials—the extent of the regions increasing with the sample size. This is exactly what happened when they varied the number of the trials as an independent variable in a supplementary experiment. That is, the statistically extracted activation peaks, rather than increasing in magnitude as the sample size increased, began to descend into the noise and eventually disappear. What had been previously accepted to be "signal" turned out to be "noise."

The significance of this startling finding is that the actual existence (and, thus, the validity) of the activation peaks becomes questionable. The brain was not responding in the form of isolated activation peaks, but as a widely distributed and generalized response. This is a very important finding because it runs counter to many of the most widely accepted postulates of current brain imaging cognitive neuroscience; namely the postulate of localized and specialized nodes that are not only anatomically but also functionally demarcated from their surround. Indeed, without activation peaks, the entire edifice of spatially localized regions associated with cognitive activity becomes questionable as an operational metaphor for brain-mind relationships. In place of sparse and localized activation areas, ever-larger and ever more widely distributed areas of the brain—up to all of it—seemed to be activated by their cognitive task. In the words of Gonzalez-Castillo et al. (2012):

> Statistically significant signal changes (sometimes as low as 0.2%) time locked with the task could be observed in almost every location of the brain.
>
> *(p. 5487)*

Although Gonzalez-Castillo and his colleagues (2012) found that there were some differences in the responses produced in different regions of the brain, they also concluded that

> under optimal noise conditions, fMRI activations extend well beyond areas of primary relationship to the task; and blood-oxygen level-dependent signal changes correlated task timing appear in over 95% of the brain for a simple visual stimulation plus attention control task.
>
> *(p. 5487)*

Another study supporting the idea that nodes may not exist and that major regions of the brain are activated if adequate tests are made was reported by Thyreau et al. (2012). They also used very large subject samples ($N = 1,326$) and reported the same general result—brain-wide distributions of statistically significant effects. Indeed, these statistically significant and widely distributed results were observed not only in gray matter, but also in the white matter of the connecting tracts in the brain in a simple passive face-viewing task.

The main point that Thyreau et al. (2012) made was that as more and more subjects were included in their analysis, that any tests of significance tend to "cross the threshold for significance however low the effect and whatever the underlying tissue may be" (p. 301). They observed that this illustrated an important difference between their work and earlier studies. As they noted,

> We obtain a wide activated pattern, far from being limited to the reasonably expected brain areas, illustrating the difference between statistical significance and practical significance.
>
> *(p. 295)*

A similar example of how repeated measures can give rise to false positive responses in an fMRI experiment has been reported by Eklund, Andersson, Josephson, Johannesson, and Knutsson (2012). They examined 1,484 fMRI brain datasets that had been previously studied to determine if there was any significant activity during cognitive rest periods. Assuming a 0.05 criterion of significance, it was expected that only 5% of these datasets should have contained any significant response peaks. Nevertheless, depending on conditions, false positive rates (accepting that significant peaks were present when they were not defined by the stimulus conditions) could range up to 70% of the datasets. Eklund et al. attributed this to a failure in the autocorrelation algorithm in the data processing package they used. However, a similar discrepancy (up to a 19% false positive rate) was also produced by an alternative data processing package. Eklund and his colleagues were conscientious in not overgeneralizing their results; nevertheless, their work also highlighted how methods rather than the subject's psychobiology could distort interpretations of fMRI data.

The implication of the Eklund et al. experiment, like those of Thyreau et al. and Gonzalez-Castillo et al., is that many reports of discrete, localized activation sites may be heavily influenced by statistical artifacts because of inadequate sample size. To put it baldly, given a complex surface or volume, peaks may randomly appear only to sink below an arbitrary criterion level as more trials are introduced into the calculation. This is due to the statistically obvious, but often overlooked, fact that even low-probability events can occur given enough repeated tests. In other words, although an experiment may be producing statistically significant findings, these false "significant" findings may be misrepresenting the actual psychobiology of the system under study.[6] This is the "fallacy of classical inference," a phenomenon in which an experiment is so overpowered that it attaches significance to even tiny effects (Friston, 2012).

Thus, all three of these experiments are making the point that rather than converging on a better estimate of sparse localized functional brain regions, increasing the sample size leads to ever more widely distributed brain regions including such unlikely places as the connecting white matter. These findings are strong arguments supporting the contention that the putative peaks appearing with small samples may be statistical artifacts rather than real biologically and cognitively significant responses and, therefore, of questionable validity. Without localized peaks of activity, no current connectionist model could survive because that whole metaphor is based on interconnected sets of *real* localized nodes.

There are two especially salient effects of conceptualizing brain responses as broadly distributed regions rather than localized nodes. First, the distribution of the amplitudes of individual neural activity peaks, as I have defined them, is random and they are independent of each other. Second, when we examine a surface such as a map of the brain, we do so from a God-like point of view that considers all locations simultaneously. This represents an experiment with many repeated measures, albeit simultaneously measured. If we concentrated on identifying the probabilistically rare large peaks, we would be led to make the error of assuming that any locations in which they occurred were correlated with the cognitive activity despite the fact that these were simply random events. This bias would result in a high level of false positives at what are essentially random locations. To the degree that these rare large peaks are randomly scattered across the brain, we would incur a large number of false positives, and this is exactly what we see in such plots as that shown in Figure 2.1.

The caveat implicit in this discussion is that because of the possible random origins of the peaks, we must take care not to be misled to associate a fortuitously large response (and the area of the brain in which it occurs) with a particular cognitive process. Thus, peaks, rather than being enhanced by the accumulation of additional data, would actually represent low probability, high amplitude, extreme values that would otherwise tend to "average out" with sufficiently large repeated measures. This demonstration also implies that the traditional $p = 0.05$ criterion level used by psychologists and equivalently low levels used by cognitive neuroscientists is far too liberal for systems as complex as those of the brain. The artifacts in this case (false positive judgments of the existence of nodes) can and do occur, and they are not discriminated against adequately by current analysis methods.

These articles and the work of Oosterwijk et al. (2012), therefore, raise serious questions about the validity of the basic idea of discrete, isolatable activation peaks. They collectively suggest that the "peaks" occurring when relatively small samples are used in an experiment may be artifacts resulting from the misuse or the inadequacy of statistical methods or from an underappreciation of the fact that unlikely outcomes can occur in any stochastic process given enough repetitions. Because brain imaging devices simultaneously examine a broad swath of the brain, the opportunity to observe one of these unlikely events is very great. As a result, many reported activation peaks might better be deemed to be false positives.

This work and the new metaphor to which it points are especially important because they provide a very different perspective on the germane organization of the brain's functions. Where the existence of localized peaks may have previously been the core postulate of MCT theory, we may now have to consider the possibility that they are just an unusual kind of noise with which our analysis techniques do not adequately deal. We may, thus, have to look upon them as invalid measures that are not measuring what they purport to be measuring. Most seriously, this line of inquiry raises questions about the entire current "nodal" metaphor of brain organization.

Other statistical errors abound that also challenge our collective ideas of the validity of brain images as either correlates or instantiations of mind. As upsetting as the invalidity of nodes may be to investigators in this field, there is currently no doubt that the possibility of our statistical analysis leading us to false positive (i.e., accepting a peak as being significantly correlated with cognition) is real and probably more prevalent than we realize. The works of Vul, Harris, Winkielman, and Pashler (2009), Vul and Kanwisher (2010), and Kriegeskorte, Simmons, Bellgowan, and Bake (2009) in which the misleading effects of "double dipping" were demonstrated are strong evidence of how we can go wrong because of a not-so-subtle misuse of the analytical techniques used to process raw data.

The problem of double dipping—the preselection of regions of interest prior to a main analysis—is not restricted to the neuroscientific problem highlighted by Vul and his colleagues. Fiedler (2011), for example, argues that this error is common through almost all forms of behavioral research in which various details of experimental design are predetermined and resulting data are subsequently analyzed using that assumption.

There are other subtle ways in which our statistical analyses can lead us astray. Bennett, Wolford, and Miller (2009), for example, have called our attention to a relatively simple artifact caused by the very large number of voxels that must be tested for statistical significance. This is another way of expressing the bias introduced by ignoring the fact that an experiment may be inadvertently overlooking the fact that a distributed surface may cryptically ignore the fact that the number of tests is larger than intended. As the number of possible tests (or regions examined) goes up (remember the significance of the response of each voxel is an individual test), the probability of false positives (asserting that a voxel is activated by a cognitive stimulus or task when it is not) also increases. According to them, it is absolutely necessary to correct the criterion p value to account for the number of tests; otherwise, large numbers of false positives would be generated.[7]

A more general criticism leading to false positives has been made by Simmons et al. (2011). They suggest that lack of constraints in the design and execution of experiments can lead to "presenting anything as significant" (p. 1359). They argue that experiments, in general, offer so many choices about such factors as subject sample size, termination points, and dealing with outliers, that "the likelihood of at least one (of many) analyses producing a false positive finding at the 5% level is necessarily greater than 5%" (p. 1359). Thus, inadequate replications and other surprisingly common statistical errors suggest that localized peaks may be illusions rather than robust phenomena.

Valid or Not, Are fMRI Responses Reliable?

The validity question will always be problematic; no matter how high the correlation, scientists of all persuasions agree that there is rarely, if ever, absolute truth and that hidden, indirect variables may sometime imitate direct causal forces. At the very least, however, scientists must be assured that the data, whatever their causal origins, are reliable before they can be used as a foundation for theory building. Reliability, therefore, is the ultimate test for the acceptance of any scientific measurement. Independent of their meaning, validity, or causal relations, reliability, consistency, and repeatability are required before phenomena can be accepted as robust data. Unreliable results should be beyond the pale of normal science.[8]

There are many factors that can influence the reliability of brain image responses during cognitive processing. Since the publication of my *New Phrenology* book (Uttal, 2001), I have repeatedly alluded to the difficulty in defining the cognitive components in this kind of research. In general, once beyond the sensory and motor representations, what constitutes an emotional, attentive, decision-making, or any other high-level cognitive process is not easy to define precisely. Nor can we guarantee that even a well-defined stimulus will actually produce the same cognitive effects from one subject to another, much less than from one experiment to another; different subjective interpretations of the meaning of even the best defined stimuli and changes due to previous experience may produce different cognitive and neural responses on the part of a subject.

The great adaptive powers of the brain also suggest that the neural response to even the most carefully constrained stimulus task may differ between what are intended to be identical experiments.

Despite the importance of tests of reliability and consistency in any scientific enterprise, but, especially in a noisy domain such as mind-brain relations, it is remarkable how little attention has been paid to the important topic of reliability. Much of brain imaging research is still in the same state as those Victorian butterfly collections; observations are simply added to an ever-expanding collection of unrelated findings in which brain activity and cognitive states are compared.

There are several unsurprising reasons why this should be the case. First, brain imaging cognitive neuroscience is, at best, only a couple of decades old. It is, therefore, a new science and may not have yet enjoyed the luxury of stable methodologies and consistent responses.

Second, the cognitive phenomena that are available for study are extremely numerous and, as previously discussed, poorly defined. Consider all of the possible cognitive activities that psychologists have studied for centuries. Even the relatively large number of cognitive neuroscientists who are using psychological taxonomies have not begun to explore the full range of possible cognitive research topics. Therefore, there has been little reason to repeat past experiments.

Third, there are the usual social pressures to make novelty as a prime criterion for publication and professional recognition. Publication in scientific journals tends to select results that are both positive and novel; studies that simply replicate or, even more seriously, reject earlier results encounter serious obstacles to publication. Furthermore, recognition by one's scientific peers depends on one's discovery of new phenomena, not just support or rejection of previous work. Prizes are not given for conclusively demonstrating that some previous result was either sound or unsound. Nor are prestigious awards recalled when previous discoveries or explanations are shown to have been wrong. Egas Moniz did not have to return his Nobel Prize when the therapeutic role of frontal lobotomies was discredited.

Fourth, it has not been widely appreciated just how difficult it is to accurately report the protocols of complex brain image experiments. Beyond the tendency to misinterpret statistical manipulations, there is always the perennial problem of simple computational errors that can lead one away from a valid theory. It is not known how widespread this problem is in cognitive neuroscience, in particular, but a suggestion that this possibility should not be overlooked has come from the work of Bakker and Wicherts (2011). They studied the misreporting of statistical results in psychology journals and found the rather disconcerting proportion of 18% of their sample of 281 articles involved errors in the statistical analyses. Even more serious than these calculation errors was that 15% of their sample of articles erred in their conclusion regarding the significance (or lack of significance) of their results.

A similar study has been carried out in the neurosciences by Nieuwenhuis, Forstmann, and Wagenmakers (2011). They were concerned about statistical tests between experimental and control animals. The problem is that comparisons of the significance of the tests for the two groups are statistically incorrect because "the differences between the significant and not significant need not itself be statistically significant." The correct strategy, therefore, is to compare "the statistical significance of the difference rather than the difference between significance levels" (p. 1105).

Having identified this common statistical problem, Nieuwenhuis and his colleagues surveyed a sample of 157 articles in prestigious neuroscience journals that were making this kind of comparison. Astonishingly, half of the 157 carried out the statistical analysis incorrectly. Other researchers (Henson, 2005; Poldrack, 2008) cited by them also specifically dealt with the same problem of comparing significance levels and found multiple instances of such interpretive errors scattered throughout the literature.

Carp (2012a), in a major review of the field, describes the vast discrepancies in reporting experimental procedures and statistical methods including the most basic information for repeating an experiment. Based on a sample of 241 reports, he asserted that,

> Many studies do not report critical methodological details with regard to experimental design, data acquisition, and analysis. Further, many studies were underpowered to detect any but the largest statistical effects. Finally, data collection and analysis methods were highly flexible across studies, with nearly as many unique analysis pipelines as there were studies in the sample.
>
> *(p. 289)*

And,

> Although many journals urge authors to describe their methods to a level of detail such that independent investigators can fully reproduce their efforts, the results described here suggest that few studies meet this criterion.
>
> *(p. 297)*

Despite situations like these, there are only a few cognitive neuroscientists who study reliability and even fewer (if any) who have explicitly adopted the role of replicator of previously reported work.[9] This is a disconcerting fact because, even to the first approximation, there are major differences between brain image findings for what are designed to be similar (enough to be considered to be repetitions) experiments no matter how well the experimental conditions are controlled.

Variability in brain images can be attributed to a very large number of possible factors, some of which are psychobiological in nature and others of which depend on the instrumentation. Not only do subjects differ from each other but also the same subject may not respond in the same way from one test to another. In dealing with such variable patterns of responses, such as those that include both an MRI magnet and a human subject, many experimental parameters may be very difficult to control. The multitude of sources of variability include such potential sources as subject movement within the magnets, state of alertness, or even how a subject interprets instructions, and many others. The following list, for example, is a portion of a list I first presented in Uttal (2013) in which I tabulated the sources of variability with which one must contend whenever one tries to compare brain imaging data from different subjects or experiments:

1. Cognitive Variability
   - Vagueness in instructions
   - Lack of stimulus control
   - Poorly defined cognitive responses
   - Variability in subject's cognitive state and strategies
   - Interference from uncontrolled cognitive states
   - Subject's affective state
   - Restricted subject diversity
   - Test-retest intervals
2. Technical Artifacts
   - Intended fluctuations in magnetic field strength in fMRI systems
   - Uncontrolled variations in field strength
   - Subject body, head, and jaw movements
   - Uncontrolled blood pressure and other orthostatic factors such as peristalsis
   - Other uncontrolled autonomic responses
   - Magnet acoustic noise
   - Equipment signal-to-noise ratios
   - Interlaboratory procedural and statistical differences
3. Decision Criteria
   - Arbitrary variations in thresholds
   - Arbitrary variations in significance criteria
   - Overemphasis on peak activations
4. Neurobiological Variability
   - Natural variability in brain responses to the same stimulus or task
   - Individual differences in brain anatomy
   - Individual differences in brain physiology
   - Inadequate brain maps
   - Inadequate language for localization

- Inadequate localization coordinates
- Fatigue and vigilance
- Variations in physiological noise with magnet strength

5. Statistical and Methodological Errors in Meta-Analyses
    - Complexity of three-dimensional statistical analyses
    - Preanalysis or inappropriate pooling of experimental data
    - Using high criterion thresholds
    - Using low criterion thresholds
    - Mixing variable thresholds or significance criteria
    - Non-normal distributions of data
    - Lack of a common metric
    - Voxel size differences between experiments
    - Different analysis methods
    - Attempting to average spatial patterns
    - Pooling nonequivalent data
    - Artificially elevating type II errors by attempts to minimize type I errors
    - Attempting to achieve significance from a pool of insignificant studies by a meta-analysis
    - Double dipping
    - Cherry-picking data

The powerful influence of whatever is the prevailing metaphor of brain organization in guiding experimental design—the current intellectual Zeitgeist—also should not be overlooked.

The theoretical possibility that each and any of these listed sources of unreliability shown in the previous list might lead to outcome variability or artifacts in brain image responses is made more plausible by examining actual empirical results from studies designed explicitly to study reliability. Specifically, although the data are still relatively sparse, there is now evidence beginning to accumulate that supports the contention that results from the following levels of data analysis are variable and inconsistent beyond acceptable limits of scientific acceptability. In the subsequent sections, I present a brief review of results bearing on this surprising conclusion emphasizing the following levels of comparison:

- Intravoxel comparisons
- Intrasubject comparisons
- Intersubject comparisons
- Interexperiment comparisons
- Meta-analytic comparisons

The full details of these comparisons are available in Uttal (2013). An abbreviated summary is presented here.

Intravoxel Comparisons

Operating at the most microneuronal level possible with an fMRI device, Nemani, Atkinson, and Thulborn (2009) examined the variability of individual voxel responses in an fMRI experiment. According to them, the size of the voxel they used "approach[es] the size of the functional unit, the cortical column, in the human primary visual cortex" (p. 1417). Their concern was with the averaging process in which multiple brain images were pooled to give a cumulative estimate of the cortical response. That is, were the voxels being averaged really describing the average activity of neurons in that voxel?

Using a particularly high resolution fMRI system, Nemani et al. (2009) examined the individual voxels from individual subjects to determine if responses were consistent from one trial to the next. Despite the fact that this was a visual perception task and that the behavioral and perceptual responses should, therefore, have remained relatively constant, they reported that there was substantial inconsistency among 40 voxel-level responses for which there were sufficiently similar experimental conditions. It was not just a matter of slight differences in the amplitude of the voxel responses but "even highly active voxels demonstrate inconsistent activation to the same repeated stimulus" (p. 1417). The variability they observed did not seem to be attributable to some kind of adaptation simply based on repetition.

This finding is interesting because it also suggests that different neural responses may encode perceptual responses even on a trial-to-trial basis. This makes the cognitive neuroscience task of finding correlations between mind and brain responses ever more difficult. Not only are there behavioral differences between subjects, but there are also differences between macroneural and (presumably) microneuronal responses from the same individual. This neural variability occurs not only in the cognitive areas of the brain but also in relatively peripheral (i.e., primary sensory cortex) regions. These discrepancies compound the usual problems of variability with a level of inconsistency that makes establishing such a relationship like shooting at a moving target. Nemani et al.'s work also implies that there may be no stable answer to the "where" question and that averaging responses is intrinsically misleading. Their results also remind us that vastly different microneuronal neuronal network states may produce identical BOLD responses because of both psychobiological variability and the various cumulative processing steps between the microneuronal and the macroneural.

Intrasubject Comparisons

Although the high level of technical sophistication of fMRI systems and the hope that individual human subjects would exhibit some kind of consistency from trial to trial may have led to the expectation of reliable responses when individual subjects were tested and retested, it turned out that this conclusion is also not, in general, supported by the empirical evidence. Given the intrinsic importance of the reliability issue, the variability of fMRI responses to cognitive stimuli from repeated tests[10] in individual subjects has been studied by an unfortunately small number of investigators. Three (Aguirre et al., 1998; McGonigle et al., 2000; and Miller et al., 2002) who did attack the problem of intrasubject variability all came to the same conclusion: Individual subjects placed in what are supposed to be identical cognitive tasks exhibit substantial day-to-day macroneural brain image variability from trial to trial. The degree of variability varies, of course, but according to Miller et al. it averages about $r = 0.5$. It is clear that any attempt to average or pool data even from a single subject results in what can be misleading attempts to define a consistent response for that subject.

Intersubject Comparisons

The variability exhibited by a single subject from trial to trial is substantial, but it is still less than the variability observed between subjects. Intersubject variability expressed as correlation between pairs of subjects is typically twice that of individual subjects compared with themselves (Miller et al., 2002).

Comparisons between brain images from different subjects provide a qualitative estimate of intersubject variability. Researchers such as Miller et al. (2002), Donovan and Miller (2008), and Poline, Thirion, Roche, and Meriaux (2010) have all shown that subjects vary among themselves to a substantial degree especially when cognitive rather than sensory and motor processes are considered. Higher order cognitive processes produce results that often have little if any overlap of the activated regions when subjects are compared. Miller et al. (2002) suggest between subject correlations in an episodic retrieval experiment are typically $r = 0.20$.

Interexperiment Comparisons

Trying to get an estimate of interexperiment variability is like counting the number of particles of sand on a beach. Examples of inconsistency in measuring brain images are evidenced by virtually every means of displaying data and every pair-wise comparison of experimental results. One of the best pieces of evidence that interexperiment variability is substantial can be seen in plots of the purported locations of activation peaks collected in preparation for a meta-analysis, an example of which was reported by Kober et al. (2008) is shown in Figure 2.1. (A variety of similar plots of widely dispersed activation sites produced by cognitive tasks can be found in Uttal, 2013). This figure plots the location of raw data—the significant activation peaks reported in a number of different experiments before the data have been pooled or meta-analyzed. The general impression is that most regions of the brain are populated with reported peaks. To extract any general conclusion of what these responses mean for localization, it has been deemed to be necessary to search for subtle, statistically defined high-density clusters of these peaks. However, in doing so, we are left with the problem—what do the excluded peaks (which were significant in their original experiments) mean?

Meta-Analytic Comparisons

In our effort to overcome poor signal-to-noise conditions and underpowered experimental designs, cognitive neuroscience has turned to cumulative statistical tools to enhance the sensitivity of our measurements. One source of the poor signal-to-noise problem we have already encountered is that too few subjects are used in a typical brain image experiment. Inadequate subject sample size is caused by simple economic pressures; it takes a considerable amount of machine time and money to run brain imaging studies and relatively few laboratories are endowed sufficiently well to be able to use an appropriately large number of subjects. This typically results in statistically low-powered experimental designs with the exception of a few studies such as those reported by Thyreau et al. (2012) and Gonzalez-Castillo et al. (2012).

There are several responses to this situation. Cognitive neuroscientists, in an effort to produce adequately powered experiments, have in the last decade or so turned to a method—meta-analysis—used in many other sciences that also confront noisy conditions and inadequate subject samples. Meta-analyses are designed to increase the statistical power of a collection of studies by pooling their individual outcomes. The idea is that the pooled results of the contributing experiments will collectively give a more accurate statement of the brain mechanisms of the cognitive process under investigation by improving the virtual power of the analysis than would any of the individual experiments.

One would expect, according to this line of logic, that, as meta-analyses are carried out and as the virtual power of the experiment increases, that two meta-analyses dealing with a common cognitive process would tend to agree more strongly than would two arbitrarily chosen experiments. Although it is difficult to quantify the degree of agreement between two meta-analyses, it seems that the expressed hope that this sequential pooling of data should result in more accurate estimates of central tendencies has not been fulfilled. Comparisons made between pairs of meta-analyses[11] (Uttal, 2013) chosen from a number of fields, however, typically showed little agreement.

Although most of the comparisons reported earlier involved only two meta-analyses, in the case of the heavily researched field of working memory, there were seven meta-analyses available to be compared. The results of these seven meta-analyses, also originally published in Uttal (2013) are presented in Table 5.1. (*BA refers to the Brodmann areas that were reported to be activated in a working memory experiment.)

TABLE 5.1 A Comparison of Seven Meta-Analyses of the Working Memory Task

BA*	Meta A	Meta B	Meta C	Meta D	Meta E	Meta F	Meta G
3							X
4				X			
6	X	X	X	X	X	X	X
7	X		X	X	X	X	X
8	X				X		
9	X		X		X		X
10	X	X	X		X	X	X
11	X						
13	X	X					X
17	X						
18	X						X
19	X	X	X	X			X
21	X			X			
22	X		X	X			
24	X					X	X
31	X						
32	X	X	X		X	X	X
37	X		X	X			
39	X						
40	X	X	X		X	X	X
44	X		X		X		X
45	X	X			X	X	X
46	X		X		X	X	
47		X				X	

(Originally published in Uttal, 2013)

* Plus scattered reports of thalamus, cerebellar, etc., activations.

The activation data in this table are taken from the following articles by column: A, Wager and Smith (2003); B, Glahn et al. (2005); C, Simmonds, Pekar, and Mostofsky (2008); D, Turkeltaub, Eden, Jones, and Zeffiro (2002); E, Owen, McMillan, Laird, and Bullmore (2005); F, Chein, Fissell, Jacobs, and Fiez (2002); G, Krain, Wilson, Arbuckle, Castellanos, and Milham (2006).

Although I propose no simple quantitative measure of the consistency of these results, it seems evident that there is a great deal of variation among the seven summarized meta-analyses concerning the brain regions associated with working memory.[12] Indeed, the only Brodmann area that was reported by all seven of the meta-analyses as being activated during working memory cognition was BA 6, a region more often associated with planning complex motor activity than with working memory (assuming that they are actually different cognitive processes). The only other brain areas common to at least six of the seven meta-analyses were, BA 10, 32, and 40. However, the specific relation of these areas to working memory is also open to question. BA 10 and BA 32 are frontal areas historically associated with cognitive activity in general and, thus, may not be specific to working memory. The functions of BA 40 are less well understood; but it is near what have traditionally been considered to be speech areas and may participate in reading tasks according to some investigators. Furthermore, there were many other subcortical regions not identified by the Brodmann nomenclature that also showed wide discrepancies among the seven meta-analyses.

Of course, this is a very rough comparison of the various areas reported as being involved in working memory. Clearly, there must have been a substantial diversity with regard to what constitutes the working memory tasks that were used as stimuli in these seven experiments. This illustrates once again the role played by inadequate definitions of cognitive processes in this type of research. The point being made here, however, is that the results of this group of seven meta-analyses do not agree well enough so that we can conclude with any assurance that any particular pattern of brain region activity is specifically encoding working memory.

What the comparisons presented throughout this section collectively show is that there is a very large amount of variability at all levels of analysis. Without some degree of consistency, the very validity of these measures is open to question and the entire edifice of brain image comparisons with cognitive processes, so laboriously constructed over the last couple of decades, may be of little help in developing a neuroreductionist theory of cognition.

5.6   Other Indications of Variability

This chapter has taken us for an excursion into what may be an emerging appreciation throughout cognitive science of what appear to be unreliable findings of questionable validity. To what can this extreme failure of an especially active field of modern science be attributed? One suggestion is that the BOLD responses produced by the fMRI methodology are simply invalid—that they are not measuring what we believe them to be measuring—they are not actually neural correlates of cognitive activity. That is, as a result of the enormous complexity of the mind-brain system and the inadequacies of our methodology, fMRI images simply may not be associable with cognitive processes in the manner currently supposed by main stream cognitive neuroscience. It is also possible that we are far too strongly influenced by what in retrospect are poorly defined iconic studies from the past; studies that misled us to expect underdetermined localization. For example, assertions that the hippocampus plays a central role in memory were originally based on early interpretations of a poorly controlled and even worse, an apparently misinterpreted surgical experiment (Scoville & Milner, 1957). Although the details were widely ignored, Scoville and Milner's original report consisted of 10 subjects, not just the iconic case of HM. Of this sample, two showed no effect; five had slight effects, and only three displayed the iconic response of short memory deficits caused by hippocampal lesions that made HM so famous. As modern research findings have accumulated, two conceptual developments emerged that cast doubt on the simple hippocampus hypothesis; first, it was appreciated that the learning role (converting short-term to long-term memory—the process known as consolidation) attributed to the hippocampus was only a part of the functions that this anatomical structure had to perform. For example, it was also discovered that it was deeply involved in spatial localization (for a review, see Eichenbaum, Dudchenko, Wood, Shapiro, & Tanila, 1999)—a discovery that led to the Nobel Prize in 2014 for three cognitive neuroscientists—John O'Keefe, May-Britt Moser, and Edvard I. Moser.[13]

Second, many other regions of the brain than the hippocampus have been subsequently shown to be involved in information storage and retrieval. Consolidation was not interfered solely by hippocampal lesions or temporal and frontal cortex lesions. The amygdala and the thalamus, as well, have also been implicated in the learning and memory storage processes. Aggleton and Sahgal (1993), for example, showed what they interpreted as a thalamic role in memory consolidation. Indeed, even the cerebellum has been implicated as participating in some simpler forms of learning such as classical conditioning (Thompson, 2005).

With the increased activity in the study of brain mechanisms of learning came increased variability in experimental results. This was a disturbing development because it differed so much from the idealized conception of what science is supposed to be accomplishing—an ever-increasing convergence on the "truth" as more and more information is pooled. In general, increases in variability raise concern about the validity of many cognitive neuroscientific studies. In this context, Lehrer (2010) discussed the general problem of the "disappearing result." He noted that there is a long history of what appear initially to be solid scientific findings (exemplified by the discovery of the "verbal overshadowing"[14] effect by Schooler and Engstler-Schooler, 1990) but that seem to progressively weaken or even disappear when they are replicated. This diminishing effect of what had been considered to be a solid effect, according to Lehrer, is most pronounced in studies of psychology and clinical pharmacology.

After showing the phenomenon of disappearing results to be a widespread effect throughout behavioral science (among others), Lehrer (2010) attributed such disappearing phenomena to a widespread constellation of factors. These included selective reporting, prejudgments of what the results should be, the misunderstanding of what statistical significance really implies, and, most important in the present context of brain imaging, that, in fact, a "lot of extraordinary scientific data are nothing but noise" (n.p.).

In such a context, it is far too easy to misinterpret what are stochastic processes and attempt to impose a fallacious kind of order on them. All of the bias sources shown in Table 5.1 contribute to distorted conclusions and errors in statistical significance. Despite what is increasingly robust evidence to the contrary, we try to force order by selecting those data that are most "significant" while ignoring the substantial proportion of the data that are classified as outliers. In doing so, we have ignored the limitations and uncertainty of statistical analysis and, quite possibly, allowed randomness, rather than causal factors, to dominate our research. As forewarned by Gonzalez-Castillo et al. (2012) and Thyreau et al. (2012), there are powerful hidden forces at work that can produce apparent order where there is none. These include inadequate sample sizes and analysis methods that are predicated on a particular assumption (e.g., localized activation peaks) about the organization of the brain.

The progressive decline in reliability of such phenomena as "verbal overshadowing" is reminiscent of the situation in cognitive neuroscience today. Despite the fact that the mix of method and preexisting theory available to us has enormous face validity (the brain is indisputatively the organ of the mind) and we are applying powerful statistical techniques that should work, there is an abundance of new empirical evidence that countervail current views of the reliability and probably the validity of brain images. Therefore, there is increasing empirical support for the argument presented here that the macroneural neural signals may well be nothing but joint artifacts of our techniques and the intrinsic complexity of the mind-brain system.

5.7   Interim Summary

This chapter summarizes some of the empirical evidence that argues against the conventional function-specific, location-dependent, macroneural theories of cognition-brain relationships. In it, I argue that progress in developing theories at this macroneural level of analysis is generally misdirected—a premise supported by a variety of newly reported empirical findings. My goal is not only to understand how this misdirection evolved in the last three decades since the functional MRI machine appeared on the cognitive neuroscience scene, but also to demonstrate that there is a corpus of empirical evidence of this misdirection.

After adding a note of precision to what constitutes a macroneural theory, I review some of the critiques that have been made of the field by Farah (2014) and suggest some responses to them. A discussion of some recent data that suggest further that the idea of localized brain nodes may be an invalid model on which to base future theories is then introduced.

Some of the strongest data challenging the macroneural approach is forthcoming from an unfortunately sparse collection of studies of reliability—the general result being that major portions of the empirical results are not replicable at any of the experimental protocol levels (voxel, intrapersonal, interpersonal, etc.) at which macroneural models operate. Thus, the most basic requirement of a theory—that its empirical foundation be solid—may not hold. The implication of the twin empirical failures of validity and reliability is that cognitive neuroscience may have to look elsewhere than the archives of macroneural data obtained from brain imaging equipment for the core of an overarching theory of mind–brain relations. Where might this alternative be found? One possibility is to emphasize the microneuronal postulates and findings of a different kind of network—that of the myriad of neurons and their interconnections that lie at a much smaller scale of magnification than is evidenced in the macroneural level of analysis. But that is another story to be told in the future.

Notes

1. I am especially concerned about the "retreat to methodology"—the ever-increasing effort to find ever-smaller and less theoretically significant phenomena.
2. By a stochastic process, I am referring to a process that is not entirely deterministic but is affected both by deterministic processes and by random processes, the latter preventing simple deterministic solutions to problems.
3. However, it must also be appreciated that all of these predecessor sciences leave their traces like fossil ideas deeply embedded in current practice. Psychosurgery is still carried out, although rarely for psychiatric disorders (most often these days for tumor removal or to control epilepsy). The roots of modern chemistry can be traced back to alchemy; astronomy to the observations of the first astrologers, and the primitive locationist theories underlying phrenology and psychosurgery still influence cognitive neuroscience.
4. The fact that the raw data—the locations of the putative peaks—were distributed over broad regions of the brain led investigators to develop techniques for determining where the activation foci were statistically densest. The next logical step was to assume that these densest regions or statistically significant clusters were the ones associated with the cognitive stimulus, thus removing us one step further from the raw data. Indeed, outlying peaks (i.e., activation areas that did meet the significance criterion for inclusion in a cluster) were simply ignored as only the most significant clusters were used to define cognitively salient brain regions. The residual problem, of course, is what is the meaning of all of the activation peaks or nodes that were not included in the densest clusters?
5. Gonzalez-Castillo and his colleagues were somewhat vague in their defining of the size and nature of their sample. They stated, "we acquired a total of 100 functional runs (i.e., 500 trials) in each of three subjects" (p. 5487). It is sufficient to note that whatever they meant by this phrase, they were dealing with an extraordinarily large sample of raw data—an amount that gave robust credibility to their conclusions and support for the idea that the nodes may be fictitious.
6. We cannot be sure exactly why this happens. Perhaps the typical 0.05 criterion is too low for highly variable experiments to probe the mind-brain relation; perhaps it is because sample sizes in this field are typically too low; perhaps it is because the whole hypothesis testing methodology used by cognitive and cognitive neuroscientists is flawed in some other fundamental way. Whatever it is, the point being made by these workers who heroically deal with such large samples is that our current analytical methods leave much to be desired and, by assuming that small samples are adequate, they may be distorting our view of the mind-brain relationship.
7. Bennett, Wolford, and Miller report that as many as 30% of the neuroimaging articles published in 2008 did not make the necessary corrections for the cryptic number of tests—a situation that could lead to many spurious results. The general point is that

sometime subtle and sometime not-so-subtle statistical phenomena can drastically distort our findings.

8. Of course, irregular, but valid, data caused by noisy conditions are possible. The problem for science in such a case is to identify the sources of noise or to find regularity in statistical terms by averaging or pooling data. Whatever data smoothing may be carried out, public replication is a sine qua non of any science. Indeed, without reliability, the validity of measures is challenged.

9. Recently, Carpenter (2012) reports that an effort to test the reliability of psychological research is being pursued by a group of psychologists under the rubric of "Open Science Collaboration." They will attempt to replicate the publications in three psychology journals and determine their reproducibility. Obviously, there is much concern about many aspects of this effort, but it would be a step forward if brought to fruition—regardless of whether they found a suitable level of reliability exists throughout the literature.

10. On the other hand, some studies (e.g., Hall et al., 1999; Peelen & Downing, 2005) have reported relatively high levels of intrasubject consistency. However, these findings have been largely associated with sensory or motor processes which, as argued repeatedly here, are more stable than the neural processes underlying cognitive processes. The conflict between these data and those of Nemani et al. may be due to the different level of analysis each represents, or it may be because the fMRI approach itself is far more flawed than is generally appreciated.

11. The research topics studied pair wise in Uttal (2013) were (1) autobiographical memory, (2) emotional face processing, (3) single-word reading, (4) N-back working memory, and (5) emotions. The reason for the selection of these pairs was simple availability—a search for relevant meta-analyses turned up very few pairs of meta-analyses that were directly comparable. None of the pairings produced similar regional identifications as measured either by common Brodmann areas or verbal designations (e.g., "supraorbital frontal cortex").

12. Although meta-analysis "A" might have seemed initially to be an artifact of too low a criterion level of significance, considering the other results discussed in this chapter it may actually have been the most correct, accurately depicting activity widely distributed over the entire brain. It is the other six that may be inaccurate by identifying only a limited number of "nodes" in each case, perhaps because of overly conservative criteria for significance. The arbitrariness of the standard "p" is, once again, highlighted by this possibility.

13. Many knowledgeable about the field feel that another important contributor to this work—Lynn Nadel—should also have been included in the award. Nadel had been a close collaborator of O'Keefe's.

14. Verbal overshadowing was defined as the inhibiting effect of attending to an object on its subsequent recognition.

6

IMPLICATIONS AND
EMERGING PRINCIPLES

> The general answer to the question asked in this book is—No! It is not possible to expect that an overarching theory of mind-brain relationships will be forthcoming from macroneural studies. The macroneural level is simply the wrong level of analysis at which to attack this profound problem. The critical micro-neuronal information that would resolve the issue is lost in records obtained from the devices that operate at the macroneural level.

This book examines the state of empirical evidence underlying macroneural network theories of mind-brain relationships at the beginning of the second decade of the 21st century. The reason for this limited perspective should be self-evident: Research in the past decade has been driven by the availability of instruments that measure the macroscopic responses of the brain. These new techniques, in particular, the fMRI, have almost completely replaced traditional techniques using electrical stimulation, surgical lesioning, or both for studying the mind-brain conundrum. Although it is anathema to many currently active cognitive scientists, the emerging generality that seems to characterize present research is that the effort to relate macroneural brain activity with cognitive processes is either premature or deeply flawed in basic principle. As this book has shown, there is increasing evidence that much of the accumulating macro-neural database is so variable as to be fairly considered to be artifacts.

The complexity of brain organization and the uncertain specification of what we mean by the various cognitive states have made this an extremely difficult field in which to conduct valid and reliable research and, thus, to develop plausible theories.

Another seductive property of this kind of brain imaging research is that it is an all-too-easy way to conduct research. Its face validity (cognition is a brain process and brain images come from the brain) is such that anyone with an MRI magnet and a stable of subjects is likely to find some kind of distinctive activity. The many conceptual, technical, statistical, and empirical problems discussed in this book, however, obscure just how difficult it is to do quality research if one's goal is to relate the cognitive and the neural domains. Thus, we do what we can do (study the cognitive functions of the brain macroneurally) when we cannot do what we should do (study the cognitive functions of the brain microneuronally).

There are many opportunities for misunderstanding and misdirection, as these complex, albeit powerful, technical methods are applied willy-nilly to the search for variable neural equivalents of ill-defined cognitive processes. Many questions remain, for example, about the validity of the BOLD response as an indicator of cognitive activity. There is a long chain of logical and inferential steps between neural codes and cognitive activity. The reasons that lead to unanswered questions are of several kinds—conceptual, technical, statistical, and empirical; collectively they raise important questions about the hope that the current approach will lead to a robust, overarching neuroreductionist theory of mind based on this technique.

Perhaps the most serious conceptual error in this field is the matter of the level of analysis—the fact that brain image measures operate at a macroneural scale that is limited to a few millimeters of resolution at best. Surprisingly, when pressed, most cognitive neuroscientists would agree that the real neurophysiological bases of cognitive are much more likely to be found at the level of microneuronal and synaptic interactions. Unfortunately, the microneuronal approach to the mind-brain problem has its own difficulties, most of which concern the combinatorial obstacles to analyzing or characterizing the myriad of neuronal types and synaptic interconnections among them. Given the combinatorial explosion associated with even small networks, that alternative may also be a dead end if the goal is to find out how the brain makes the mind.

This book presents a discussion of the many issues that challenge the utility of brain images as precursors to explanatory theories. I now sum up what I have learned from my studies in the form of a set of emerging principles that seem to express the state of current cognitive neuroscience. The summed total of this list is what I believe to be a modern metaphor for cognitive neuroscience. It is by no means a "theory" or even a "prototheory," but, instead, a point of view or an opinion about where we are today with regard to this overwhelming important problem:

1. The basic question of modern cognitive neuroscience is to answer the question, how does the brain make the mind?
2. The primary ontological postulate underlying this question is that mental activity, in all of its manifestations, is neither nothing more nor nothing less than a function of the brain.
3. However, even if one accepts without question the ontological postulate of mind-brain equivalence, there are profound epistemological limits on what

we can learn about the neural origins of cognition. These arise mainly from the complexity of the problems faced by cognitive neuroscientists.

4. Potential solutions to the basic question are unifying and integrating statements we call theories. Macroneural theories come in many kinds, virtually all of which are inadequate prototheories that finesse or otherwise ignore the main issue of mind-brain neuroreductionism.

5. There are some successes, however. We do have good understanding of the sensory and motor transmission codes because topological information is preserved at the relatively peripheral levels at which this kind of information enters or leaves the brain and in the primary sensory and motor areas. However, this does not mean that high-level cognitive processes are equally well understood or are likely to be equally well understood in the foreseeable future.

6. There are several levels of analysis at which the mind-brain problem can be studied. These range from the microneuronal level of (cellular) networks to the macroneural, cumulative macroscopic images produced by brain imaging technology. Each tool stimulates its own variety of theory or metaphor.

7. Relatively "solid" experimental findings often have a tendency to disappear when replicated. Indeed, exact replication is rare (1) because of a lack of professional reward (novelty is a key to publication success), (2) practical limits on reporting methods (it is difficult to fully report complex experimental protocols), or (3) different analysis trajectories produce different results.

8. The current most popular macroneural connectionist theory (MCT) of brain correlates of mind is based on a postulate of some kind of localized, function-specific nodes, peaks, or activation regions.

9. Recent brain image data, however, suggest that localized activation sites or nodes may well be artifacts of low power experiments or inadequate sample sizes.

10. It now appears that a widely dispersed (i.e., broadly distributed) set of brain regions are more likely to be encoding a given cognitive process rather than single or a few locations. This distribution may be as broad as the entire brain. That is, most of the brain may be involved in the representation of any cognitive process.

11. Current analytic techniques suggest that brain regions cannot be function-specific. Instead, any region can participate in many different cognitive processes. Similarly, the same cognitive process can be represented by different brain regions from one experiment to another. For this reason, it is impossible to decide what cognitive process is underway from an examination of neural activity. Therefore, brain images are not likely to "read" the mind beyond the applications that use topological constancies in the periphery.

12. As in any other science, there are many other social, economic, and historical forces at work that predispose us to accept questionable data and implausible theories as putative explanations of the relation between the brain and

cognition. The mind-brain problem is particularly susceptible to these forces because of its complexity and social relevance.

13. Formal mathematics can help to filter out the implausible from the plausible but cannot robustly discriminate between alternative reductive theories (either neural or cognitive) of cognition, many of which may be sufficient to describe system behavior, but none of which can be demonstrated to be necessary and unique.

14. Similarly, all behaviors, introspective reports of experiences, and models of all kinds are neutral with regard to underlying mechanisms. For example, no matter how precise, the behavioral description of an "experience" cannot, in principle, offer any clue to the neural mechanisms that account for that cognition.

15. Criteria such as elegance, simplicity, or predictability may be irrelevant in selecting the best theory of mind-brain relations because of the redundancy of the neural mechanism and underdetermination of the data obtained in even the best designed experiments.

16. One of the most challenging problems in this field continues to be the inadequate definition and control of cognitive states used as independent variables in cognitive neuroscience experiments. The cognitive response to a stimulus, rather than the stimulus itself, is the true independent variable. As a result, there is an inevitable lack of control of the salient independent variables used in brain imaging experiments.

17. There is no a priori reason that the component "faculties," "cognitive processes," and "modules" of the taxonomies used by psychologists to define cognitive processes should map in any direct way onto brain mechanisms. That is, the taxonomy of cognitive modules used by psychologists need not overlap with the dimensions of brain activity. It is likely that, once beyond peripheral sensory and motor codes, symbolic or nonisomorphic properties or dimensions instantiate cognitive properties or dimensions in the brain.

18. There has been a steady historical progression of the kinds of data our experiments are producing. The steps in this progression include the following:
    - Single localized nodes encoding specific functions (Phrenology and neophrenology)
    - Multiple, but still localized and independent, regions (Early Macroneural Connectionist Theories—MCT)
    - Interconnected, multiple, localized regions (Recent MCT)
    - Broadly distributed responses without specific localization

19. At each stage in this history, different metaphors, if not theories, have been invoked to describe findings. There is a historical trend toward more and more holistic interpretations stimulated by this progression from isolated, single function nodes to involvement of the whole brain.

20. Macroneural imaging data associated with cognitive processes tend to be inconsistent and unreliable at all levels of analysis. This includes intravoxel, intrasubject, intersubject, interexperiment, and meta-analysis levels.

21. There is no a priori reason to expect that the system should exactly replicate the neural representations of a cognitive process from one trial to the next. This variability, which may also be called "adaptability," is an important source of human quality of life. It is, however, an albatross around the neck of any cognitive neuroscientist who aspires to produce a stable overarching theory of mind-brain relations.

22. The extent of this variability remains uncertain. Much of the data collected is never exactly replicated, nor can they be given the many possible analytic methods that can be used to analyze raw data. Furthermore, most studies typically do not report the conditions of an experiment sufficiently well for the experiment to be exactly repeated.

23. Different analytical techniques often produce different empirical results. This variability is the result of a very large number of sources of bias and misinterpretation that can affect the outcome of experiments.

24. Statistical considerations dictate that even relatively unlikely responses occasionally occur should enough tests be carried out. With the very large number of simultaneously observed response sites on the brain, a momentary, but brain-wide, sampling (as exemplified by the brain image technology) is likely to detect some kind of low probability, but elevated, response someplace on the brain. As sample sizes or the number of repeated measures increases, significance can be attributed to ever smaller effects, thus further enhancing the false positive rate. This is a major source of the misidentification of putative activation peaks.

25. False positive responses are often interpreted as nodes or localized activation peaks whose extent depends on arbitrary thresholds set by the experimenter.

26. Many other sources of bias affect brain imaging experiments. Recent work suggests that nodes or activation sites may actually be statistical artifacts produced by small sample sizes, inadequately powered experiments, and statistical tests that prejudge the existence of the peaks or nodes.

27. The validity of the brain image responses is opened to question by the abundance of false positives (caused by statistical and computational errors) that permeate the field.

28. When one plots raw data (subsequently to be pooled for use in meta-analyses), activation nodes are observed over most of the brain. It is only when meta-analytical statistical tests are applied that a reduced number of clusters consisting of multiple nodes emerge. This may be an artifact of poor signal-to-noise ratios; however, it also raises questions about the biological reality of the nodes themselves. If nodes or localized activation areas do not exist, than much of modern thought about mind-brain relations becomes dubious.

29. It seems increasingly likely that the nodes observed in many brain images are actually nonspecific responses of multifactorial, multidimensional, nearly random systems to which we have attached a fictitious kind of order.

30. The most likely theory or metaphor available to us currently is that the brain mechanisms underlying cognitive processes are organized in a broadly distributed manner whose microneuronal complexity is so great that it is invulnerable to any formal analysis. Searching for the psychoneural equivalent of cognition may, therefore, be a fruitless task and providing an overarching theory may be impossible. This does not mean that we may not make other unexpected discoveries about the brain in our studies with these systems. However, the great mind-brain question itself is likely to remain a riddle far into the future with neither macroneural nor microneuronal approaches able to untie the World-Knot.

In summary, the conclusion to this study of current mind-brain theory is that developing robust, plausible, valid, and reliable macroneural theories is going to be an enormously difficult scientific task for as far into the future as we can see. However, no one can predict the remote future and perhaps someday a cognitive neuroscientist "Einstein" might appear on the scene who will give us some new insight into the basic nature of the problem. Nevertheless, at the moment, there is no sign of progress towards an overarching theoretical solution.

It is fair to ask then—if not the macroneural tone set by functional brain imaging, what then should we do? It is important to reiterate a point that often gets overlooked in the negative critique that is presented here—the MRI device is one of the major developments of modern science contributing to modern medicine and technology in ways that can hardly be imagined. It is the tool *par excellence* for studies of the anatomy and biochemistry of the brain and many other organs of the body. No one can possibly argue in any rational way against this vital technology and its many contributions to human welfare and science. However, its great failure resides in what some of us see as its misapplication to the problems of cognitive psychology. For the many reasons that have been reviewed here, its role in cognitive neuroscience must be considered with great care. (A curious development suggesting that such a reconsideration is actually going on in cognitive neuroscience is that there appears, on a purely intuitive basis, to be a reduction in the number of articles being published in which psychological and neural responses are being compared. Brain imaging seems now to be returning to its anatomical and physiological roots.)

Progress in mind-brain theory is constrained by two factors: (1) The overwhelming amount of information arising from the combinatorial complexity of the brain when viewed from the microneuronal point of view, and (2) the actual loss of information caused by pooling and accumulation at many levels when viewed from the macroneural point of view. These factors do not bode well for the emergence of comprehensive theory in the foreseeable future at any level.

No one can say if these barriers are impenetrable or merely temporary obstacles to the development of an overarching theory. Perhaps we will have to join the epistemologists and admit, much to our disdain, that the mind-brain problem is unsolvable. I hate to end this book on such a negative note; however, just as we are now in agreement that the development of a perpetual motion machine is impossible, perhaps also we should consider more deeply some of the hints that an overarching solution to the mind-brain problem is also going to be beyond our reach. If so—so be it—there is plenty for both neuroscientists and psychologists to do without searching for a false and elusive neuroreductionism. Unfortunately, the MCT approach seems to be unfruitful in its present form although its difficulties are of principle, not of practice. Major breakthroughs are desperately needed if we are to ever understand how our material minds make our intangible mental processes.

Given these difficulties and challenges to the current Zeitgeist concerning the relation between the cognitive and the neural, where do we stand now with regard to the prevailing metaphor? The most likely answer to this question is that, despite the lack of supporting empirical evidence, it is the Hebbian microneuronal network that is the most plausible current metaphor for the mind-brain relation. However, the practical difficulties in studying these tiny neuronal networks are also profound and may not be surmountable. They do, however, deserve more attention; this is what I plan for the next book in this series.

Added Note

The general idea behind macroneuronal theories of cognition is that by appropriately activating some aspect of cognition, we can localize regions of the brain that are in some way responsible for coding that cognitive process. There is, however, a related idea that is based on the inverse of this idea—namely that we can stimulate certain regions of the brain to manipulate cognitive processes. In the first case, we are searching for the brain locations associated with predefined cognitive states. In the second case, we are assuming that certain brain areas are related to certain cognitive states and then attempting to manipulate those cognitions by stimulating the brain locales with electrical stimuli. Both approaches are based on the same fundamental premise—namely that cognitive processes are mediated by specific macroscopic brain locations.

Work using transcranial Direct Current Stimulation (tDCS), for example, has blossomed in the last decade with suggestions that electrical stimulation of the brain can have profound effects on cognitive functions and psychiatric problems of one kind or another. Dozens if not hundreds of reports now purport to document the psychological effects of electrical stimuli directly applied to the brain. Like many other enthusiastic applications of new technologies, it now seems that what seem to be a plethora of positive effects may actually be little more than random noise. An Australian investigator by the name of Jared Horvath has reviewed and statistically analyzed large samples of tDCS experiments. In two articles (Horvath, Forte, & Carter, 2015a, 2015b), he and his colleagues concluded that there are no reliable effects of this kind of electrical stimuli on cognition. The single exception to this general result is that motor twitches, not surprisingly since the stimuli were being applied to motor areas of the brain, varied with tDCS stimulation.

Horvath, Carter and Forte (2014) went on to suggest that this poor reliability could be accounted for by five types of inadequate controls:

1. Intersubject variability
2. Intrasubject variability
3. Absence of sham stimulation and blind analysis techniques
4. Motor and cognitive interference
5. Controls for physical nature of the direct current stimuli

When examined in the light of the equally poor controls and variable results obtained with fMRI approach, this critique speaks strongly to the idea that macroneural theories, so widespread in current cognitive neuroscience, are inadequate.

REFERENCES

Adler, K. (2007). *The lie detectors: A history of American deception*. New York: Free Press.

Aflalo, T. N., & Graziano, M.S.A. (2011). Organization of the macaque extrastriate visual cortex re-examined using the principle of spatial continuity of function. *Journal of Neurophysiology, 105*(1), 305–320.

Aggleton, J. P., & Sahgal, A. (1993). The contribution of the anterior thalamic nuclei to anterograde amnesia. *Neuropsychologia, 31*(10), 1001–1019.

Aguirre, G. K., Zarahn, E., & D'Esposito, M. (1998). The variability of human, BOLD hemodynamic responses. *NeuroImage, 8*(4), 360–369.

Aldrich, J. (1995). Correlations genuine and spurious in Pearson and Yule. *Statistical Science, 10*(4), 364–376.

Alivisatos, A. P., Chun, M.Y., Church, G. M., Deisseroth, K., Donoghue, J. P., Greenspan, R. J., . . . Yuste, R. (2013). The Brain Activity Map. *Science, 339*(6125), 1284–1285.

Anderson, C. M., & Craik, F.I.M. (1974). Effect of a concurrent task on recall from primary memory. *Journal of Verbal Learning and Verbal Behavior, 13*(1), 107–113.

Anderson, R. B., & Tweney, R. D. (1997). Artifactual power curves in forgetting. *Memory & Cognition, 25*(5), 724–730.

Andreski, S. (1972). *Social sciences as sorcery*. London: Deutsch.

Ashby, F. G., Ennis, J. M., & Spiering, B. J. (2007). A neurobiological theory of automaticity in perceptual categorization. *Psychological Review, 114*, 632–656.

Ashby, F. G., & Maddox, W. T. (2005). Human category learning. *Annual Review of Psychology, 56*, 149–178.

Aue, T., Lavelle, L. A., & Cacioppo, J. T. (2009). Great expectations: What can fMRI research tell us about psychological phenomena? *International Journal of Psychophysiology, 73*(1), 10–16.

Baddeley, A. (2003). Working memory: Looking back and looking forward. *Nature Reviews Neuroscience, 4*(10), 829–839.

Baddeley, A. D., & Hitch, G.J.L. (1974). Working memory. In G. A. Bower (Ed.), *The psychology of learning and motivation: Advances in research and theory* (Vol. 8, pp. 47–89). New York: Academic Press.

Bakan, D. (1966). The test of significance in psychological research. *Psychological Bulletin, 66*(6), 423–437.

Bakker, M., & Wicherts, J. M. (2011). The (mis)reporting of statistical results in psychology journals. *Behavior Research Methods, 43*(3), 666–678.

Bannister, D. (1968). The myth of physiological psychology. *Bulletin of the British Psychological Society, 21*, 229–231.

Barrett, L. F. (2011). Bridging token identity theory and supervenience theory through psychological construction. *Psychological Inquiry, 22*(2), 115–127.

Barrett, L. F., & Satpute, A. B. (2013). Large-scale brain networks in affective and social neuroscience: towards an integrative functional architecture of the brain. *Current Opinion in Neurobiology, 23*(3), 361–372.

Bennett, C. M., Wolford, G. L., & Miller, M. B. (2009). The principled control of false positives in neuroimaging. *Social Cognitive and Affective Neuroscience, 4*(4), 417–422.

Berger, H. (1929). Uber das electroenkephalogramm de menschem. *Archiv für Psychiatrie Nervenkranken, 87*, 527–570.

Bernheim, B. D. (2009). On the potential of neuroeconomics: A critical but hopeful appraisal. National Bureau of Economic Research Paper Series (Working Paper 13954). Cambridge, MA.

Brambilla, P., Hardan, A., di Nemi, S. U., Perez, J., Soares, J. C., & Barale, F. (2003). Brain anatomy and development in autism: review of structural MRI studies. *Brain Research Bulletin, 61*(6), 557–569.

Breasted, J. H. (1930). The Edwin Smith Surgical Papyrus. *University of Chicago Oriental Institute Publications* (Vol. 3–4). Chicago: University of Chicago.

Broadbent, D. E. (1958). *Perception and communication.* New York: Pergamon Press.

Broca, P. (1861). *Bulletin de la societe'francaise d'anthorpologie, 2*, 235–238.

Brodmann, K. (1909). *Vergleichende Lokalisationlehre der Grosshirnrinde in ihrenPrinzipen dargestellt auf Grund des Zellenbaues.* Leipzig: J. A. Barth.

Brown, P. K., & Wald, G. (1964). Visual pigments in single rods + cones of human retina—direct measurements reveal mechanisms of human night + color vision. *Science, 144*(3614), 45–52.

Bullmore, E., & Sporns, O. (2009). Complex brain networks: Graph theoretical analysis of structural and functional systems. *Nature Reviews Neuroscience, 10*(4), 186–198.

Bundesen, C., Habekost, T., & Kyllingsbaek, S. (2005). A neural theory of visual attention: Bridging cognition and neurophysiology. *Psychological Review, 112*(2), 291–328.

Cajal, S.R.Y. (1900). *Die Sehrinde.* Leipzig: J. A. Barth.

Carp, J. (2012a). The secret lives of experiments: Methods reporting in the fMRI literature. *NeuroImage, 63*, 289–300.

Carp, J. (2012b). On the plurality of (methodological) worlds: Estimating the analytic flexibility of fMRI experiments. *Frontiers in Neuroscience, 6*, 1–13.

Carpenter, S. (2012). Psychology's bold initiative. *Science, 335*, 1558–1561.

Chein, J. M., Fissell, K., Jacobs, S., & Fiez, J. A. (2002). Functional heterogeneity within Broca's area during verbal working memory. *Physiology & Behavior, 77*(4–5), 635–639.

Chouinard, P. A., & Goodale, M. A. (2010). Category-specific neural processing for naming pictures of animals and naming pictures of tools: An ALE meta-analysis. *Neuropsychologia, 48*(2), 409–418.

Churchland, P.M. (1981). Eliminative materialism and the propositional attitudes. *Journal of Philosophy, 78*(2), 67–90.

Clarke, F. R. (1957). Constant-ratio rule for confusion matrices in speech communication. *Journal of the Acoustical Society of America, 29*(6), 715–720.

Coltheart, M. (2006). What has functional neuroimaging told us about the mind (so far)? *Cortex, 42*(3), 323–331.

Coltheart, M. (2010). What is functional neuroimaging for? In S. J. Hanson & S. M. Bunzi (Eds.), *Foundation issues in human brain mapping.* Cambridge, MA: MIT Press.

Coltheart, M. (2013). How can functional neuroimaging inform cognitive theories? *Perspectives on Psychological Science, 8*(1), 98–103.

Cooley, J. W., & Tukey, J. W. (1965). An algorithm for machine calculation of complex Fourier series. *Mathematics of Computation, 19*(90), 297-&.

Costafreda, S. G., Fu, C.H.Y., Lee, L., Everitt, B., Brammer, M. J., & David, A. S. (2006). A systematic review and quantitative appraisal of fMRI studies of verbal fluency: Role of the left inferior frontal gyrus. *Human Brain Mapping, 27*(10), 799–810.

Cummins, R. (1983). *The nature of psychological explanation.* Cambridge, MA: MIT Press.

de Garis, H., Chen, S., Goertzel, B., & Lian, R.T. (2010). A world survey of artificial brain projects, Part I: Large-scale brain simulations. *Neurocomputing, 74*(1–3), 3–29.

Deco, G., Jirsa, V. K., Robinson, P. A., Breakspear, M., & Friston, K. J. (2008). The dynamic brain: From spiking neurons to neural masses and cortical fields. *PLOS Computational Biology, 4*(8).

Delgado, M. R., Miller, M. M., Inati, S., & Phelps, E. A. (2005). An fMRI study of reward-related probability learning. *NeuroImage, 24*(3), 862–873.

DeValois, R. L., Abramov, I., & Jacobs, G. H. (1966). Analysis of response patterns of LGN cells. *Journal of the Optical Society of America, 56*(7), 966–977.

Dietrich, E., & Hardcastle, V.G. (2005). *Sisyphus's boulder: Consciousness and the limits of the knowable.* Amsterdam: John Benjamins.

Di Giovanni, G., & Shi, W. X. (2009). Effects of scopolamine on dopamine neurons in the substantia nigra: Role of the pedunculopontine tegmental nucleus. *Synapse, 63*(8), 673–680.

Donovan, C. L., & Miller, M. B. (2008, December 1–4). *An investigation of individual variability in brain activity during episodic encoding and retrieval.* Paper presented at the 26th Army Science Conference, Orlando, FL.

Dyson, F. W., Eddington, A. S., & Davidson, C. (1920). A determination of the deflection of light by the sun's gravitational field, from observations made at the total eclipse of 29 May 1919. *Philosophical Transactions of the Royal Society of London 220A,* 291–333.

Eichenbaum, H., Dudchenko, P., Wood, E., Shapiro, M., & Tanila, H. (1999). The hippocampus, memory, and place cells: Is it spatial memory or a memory space? *Neuron, 23*(2), 209–226.

Eklund, A., Andersson, M., Josephson, C., Johannesson, M., & Knutsson, H. (2012). Does parametric fMRI analysis with SPM yield valid results? An empirical study of 1484 rest datasets. *NeuroImage, 61*(3), 565–578.

Ekstrom, A. (2010). How and when the fMRI BOLD signal relates to underlying neural activity: The danger in dissociation. *Brain Research Reviews, 62,* 233–244.

Ekstrom, A., Suthana, N., Millett, D., Fried, I., & Bookheimer, S. (2009). Correlation between BOLD fMRI and theta-band local field potentials in the human hippocampal area. *Journal of Neurophysiology, 101*(5), 2668–2678.

Farah, M. J. (2008). A picture is worth a thousand words. *Journal of Cognitive Neuroscience, 21,* 623–624.

Farah, M. J. (2014). Brain images, babies, and bathwater: Critiquing critiques of functional neuroimaging. *Hastings Center Report, 44,* S19–S30.

Farah, M. J., & Hook, C. J. (2013). The seductive allure of "seductive allure." *Perspectives on Psychological Science, 8*(1), 88–90.

Farrow, T.F.D., Jones, S. C., Kaylor-Hughes, C. J., Wilkinson, I. D., Woodruff, P.W.R., Hunter, M. D., & Spence, S. A. (2011). Higher or lower? The functional anatomy of perceived allocentric social hierarchies. *NeuroImage, 57*(4), 1552–1560.

Feigl, H. (1958). The mental and the physical. *Minnesota Studies in the Philosophy of Science, 2,* 370–497.

Fiedler, K. (2011). Voodoo correlations are everywhere—not only in neuroscience. *Perspectives on Psychological Science, 6*(2), 163–171.

Fodor, J. A. (1983). *The modularity of mind.* Cambridge MA: MIT Press.

Fox, C. R., & Poldrack, R. A. (2009). Prospect theory and the brain. In P. Glimcher, C. Camerea, E. Fehr, & R. A. Poldrack (Eds.), *Neuroeconomics: Decision making and the brain* (pp. 145–173). London: Elsevier.

Freedman, D. J., Riesenhuber, M., Poggio, T., & Miller, E. K. (2003). A comparison of primate prefrontal and inferior temporal cortices during visual categorization. *Journal of Neuroscience, 23*(12), 5235–5246.

Friston, K. (2012). Ten ironic rules for non-statistical reviewers. *NeuroImage, 61*(4), 1300–1310.

Friston, K. J. (1994). Functional and effective connectivity in neuroimaging: A synthesis. *Human Brain Mapping, 2,* 56–78.

Friston, K. J., Ashburner, J., Kiebel, K., Nichols, T., & Penny, W. D. (2007). *Statistical parametric mapping : The analysis of functional brain images* (1st ed.). Amsterdam and Boston: Elsevier/ Academic Press.

Friston, K. J., & Price, C. J. (2011). Modules and brain mapping. *Cognitive Neuropsychology, 28*(3–4), 241–250.

Friston, K. J., Price, C. J., Fletcher, P., Moore, C., Frackowiak, R. S. J., & Dolan, R. J. (1996). The trouble with cognitive subtraction. *Neuroimage, 4*(2), 97–104.

Friston, K. J., Rotshtein, P., Geng, J. J., Sterzer, P., & Henson, R. N. (2006). A critique of functional localisers. *NeuroImage, 30*(4), 1077–1087.

Fumagalli, R. (2010). The disunity of neuroeconomics. *Journal of Economic Methodology, 17,* 119–131.

Gall, F. J., & Spurzheim, J. C. (1808). Recherches sur le systeme nerveux en general et sur celui du cerveau en particulier. *Academie de Sciences, Paris, Memoirs.*

Gallistel, C. R. (2009). The neural mechanisms that underlie decision making. In P. Glimcher, C. Camerea, E. Fehr, & R. A. Poldrack (Eds.), *Neuroeconomics: Decision making and the brain* (pp. 419–424). Amsterdam: Academic Press.

Gerstner, W., Sprekeler, H., & Deco, G. (2012). Theory and simulation in neuroscience. *Science, 338*(6103), 60–65.

Glahn, D.C., Ragland, J. D., Abramoff, A., Barrett, J., Laird, A. R., Bearden, C. E., & Velligan, D. I. (2005). Beyond hypofrontality: A quantitative meta-analysis of functional neuroimaging studies of working memory in schizophrenia. *Human Brain Mapping, 25*(1), 60–69.

Glimcher, P. (2009). Choice: Toward a standard back–pocket model. In P. Glimcher, C. F. Camerer, E. Fehr, & R. A. Poldrack (Eds.), *Neuroeconomics: Decision making and the brain.* London: Academic Press.

Glimcher, P. W., Camerer, C. F., Fehr, E., & Poldrack, R. A. (Eds.). (2009). *Neuroeconomics: Decision making and the brain.* London: Academic Press.

Goertzel, B., Lian, R. T., Arel, I., de Garis, H., & Chen, S. (2010). World survey of artificial brains, Part II: Biologically inspired cognitive architectures. *Neurocomputing, 74*(1–3), 30–49.

Gonzalez-Castillo, J., Saad, Z. S., Handwerker, D. A., Inati, S. J., Brenowitz, N., & Bandettini, P. A. (2012). Whole-brain, time-locked activation with simple tasks revealed with massive averaging and model-free analysis. *Proceedings of the National Academy of Sciences of the United States of America, 109*, 5487–5492.

Greicius, M. D., Krasnow, B., Reiss, A. L., & Menon, V. (2003). Functional connectivity in the resting brain: A network analysis of the default mode hypothesis. *Proceedings of the National Academy of Sciences of the United States of America, 100*(1), 253–258.

Gul, F., & Pesendorfer, W. (2008). The case for mindless economics. In A. Caplin & A. Schotter (Eds.), *The foundations of positive and normative economics: A handbook* (pp. 3–41). Oxford: Oxford University Press.

Guthrie, E. R. (1946). Psychological facts and psychological theory. *Psychological Bulletin, 43*(1), 1–20.

Hall, D. A., Haggard, M. P., Akeroyd, M. A., Palmer, A. R., Summerfield, A. Q., Elliott, M. R., . . . Bowtell, R. W. (1999). "Sparse" temporal sampling in auditory fMRI. *Human Brain Mapping, 7*(3), 213–223.

Hanson, S. J., & Halchenko, Y. O. (2008). Brain reading using full brain support vector machines for object recognition: There is no "face" identification area. *Neural Computation, 20*, 486–503.

Harary, F. (1969). *Graph theory*. Reading, MA: Addison-Wesley.

Harrison, G. W. (2008). Neuroeconomics: A critical reconsideration. *Economics and Philosophy, 24*(3), 303–344.

Haxby, J. V. (2010). Multivariate pattern analysis of fMRI data: High-dimensional spaces for neural and cognitive representations. In S. J. Hanson & M. Bunzl (Eds.), *Foundational issues in human brain mapping* (pp. 55–68). Cambridge, MA: MIT Press.

Haynes, J. D., & Rees, G. (2005). Predicting the orientation of invisible stimuli from activity in human primary visual cortex. *Nature Neuroscience, 8*(5), 686–691.

Hebb, D. O. (1949). *The organization of behavior: A neuropsychological theory*. New York: Wiley.

Heil, J. (2003). Mental causation. In S. P. Stich & T. A. Warfield (Eds.), *The Blackwell guide to the philosophy of mind* (pp. 213–234). Malden, MA: Blackwell.

Hempel, C. G. (1965). *Aspects of scientific explanation*. New York: Free Press.

Hennig, W. (1966). *Phylogenetic systematics*. Urbana: University of Illinois Press.

Henson, R. (2005). What can functional neuroimaging tell the experimental psychologist? *Quarterly Journal of Experimental Psychology Section A: Human Experimental Psychology, 58*(2), 193–233.

Henson, R. (2006). What has (neuro)psychology told us about the mind (so far)? A reply to Coltheart (2006). *Cortex, 42*(3), 387–392.

Henson, R. N. (2011). How to discover modules in mind and brain: The curse of non-linearity, and blessing of neuroimaging. A comment on Sternberg (2011) [Commentary]. *Cognitive Neuropsychology, 28*(3–4), 209–223.

Hesse, M. (1967). Laws and theories. In P. Edwards (Ed.), *The encyclopedia of philosophy*. New York: Macmillan.

Hilgetag, C. C., O'Neill, M. A., & Young, M. P. (1996). Indeterminate organization of the visual system. *Science, 271*(5250), 776–777.

Hodgkin, A. L., & Huxley, A. F. (1952). A quantitative description of membrane current and its application to conduction and excitation in nerve. *Journal of Physiology–London, 117*(4), 500–544.

Horvath, J. C., Carter, O., & Forte, J. D. (2014). Transcranial direct current stimulation: Five important issues we aren't discussing (but probably should be). [Review]. *Front Syst Neurosci, 8*, 2.

Horvath, J. C., Forte, J. D., & Carter, O. (2015a). Evidence that transcranial direct current stimulation (tDCS) generates little-to-no reliable neurophysiologic effect beyond

MEP amplitude modulation in healthy human subjects: A systematic review. *Neuropsychologia, 66*, 213–236.

Horvath, J. C., Forte, J. D., & Carter, O. (2015b). Quantitative review finds no evidence of cognitive effects in healthy populations from single-session Transcranial Direct Current Stimulation (tDCS). *Brain Stimulation, 8*(2), 535–550.

Houghton, G., Tipper, S. P., Weaver, B., & Shore, D. I. (1996). Inhibition and interference in selective attention: Some tests of a neural network model. *Visual Cognition, 3*(2), 119–164.

Ioannidis, J.P.A. (2005). Why most published research findings are false. *PLOS Medicine, 2*(8), 696–701.

Ioannidis, J.P.A., & Khoury, M. J. (2011). Improving validation practices in "omics" research. *Science, 334*, 1230–1232.

Iturria-Medina, Y., Sotero, R. C., Canales-Rodriguez, E. J., Aleman-Gomez, Y., & Melie-Garcia, L. (2008). Studying the human brain anatomical network via diffusion-weighted MRI and Graph Theory. *NeuroImage, 40*(3), 1064–1076.

Javitt, D. C., Spencer, K. M., Thaker, G. K., Winterer, G., & Hajos, M. (2008). Neurophysiological biomarkers for drug development in schizophrenia. *Nature Reviews Drug Discovery, 7*(1), 68–83.

Johnson, M. H. (2005). The development of visual attention. In M. Gazzaniga (Ed.), *The Cognitive Neurosciences* (pp. 753–747). Cambridge MA: MIT.

Jones, L. M., Fontanni, A., & Katz, D. B. (2006). Gustatory processing: A dynamic systems approach. *Current Opinion in Neurobiology, 16*, 420–428.

Kaas, J. H. (2004). Neuroanatomy is needed to define the "organs" of the brain. *Cortex, 40*, 207–208.

Kahneman, D. (2009). Remarks on neuroeconomics. In P. Glimcher, C. Camerea, E. Fehr, & R. A. Poldrack (Eds.), *Neuroeconomics: Decision making and the brain* (pp. 523–526). Amsterdam: Academic Press.

Kahneman, D., & Tversky, A. (1979). Prospect theory: An analysis of decision under risk. *Econometrica, 47*(2), 263–291.

Kamitani, Y., & Tong, F. (2005). Decoding the visual and subjective contents of the human brain. *Nature Neuroscience, 8*(5), 679–685.

Karp, R. M. (1986). Combinatorics, complexity, and randomness. *Communications of the ACM, 29*(2), 98–109.

Kennard, M. A. (1955). Effect of bilateral ablation of cingulate area on behaviour of cats. *Journal of Neurophysiology, 18*(2), 159–169.

Killeen, P. R. (1994). Mathematical principles of reinforcement. *Behavioral and Brain Sciences, 17*(1), 105–135.

Killeen, P. R. (2001). The four causes of behavior. *Current Directions in Psychological Science, 10*(4), 136–140.

Killeen, P. R. (2005). Tea-tests. *The General Psychologist, 40*, 16–19.

Klein, C. (2011). Images are not the evidence in neuroimaging. *British Journal for the Philosophy of Science, 61*, 265–278.

Kober, H., Barrett, L. F., Joseph, J., Bliss-Moreau, E., Lindquist, K., & Wager, T. D. (2008). Functional grouping and cortical-subcortical interactions in emotion: A meta-analysis of neuroimaging studies. *NeuroImage, 42*(2), 998–1031.

Koch, C. (2012). Modular biological complexity. *Science, 337*, 531–532.

Koch, C., & Greenfield, S. (2007). How does consciousness happen? *Scientific American, 297*(4), 76–83.

Krain, A. L., Wilson, A.M., Arbuckle, R., Castellanos, F.X., & Milham, M. P. (2006). Distinct neural mechanisms of risk and ambiguity: A meta-analysis of decision-making. *NeuroImage, 32*(1), 477–484.

Kriegeskorte, N., Simmons, W. K., Bellgowan, P.S.F., & Baker, C. I. (2009). Circular analysis in systems neuroscience: The dangers of double dipping. *Nature Neuroscience, 12*(5), 535–540.

Kuhn, T. S. (1962). *The structure of scientific revolutions.* Chicago: University of Chicago Press.

Lambdin, C. (2012). Significance tests as sorcery: Science is empirical—significance tests are not. *Theory & Psychology, 22*(1), 67–90.

Langers, R. M., & van Dijk, P. (2011). Robustness of intrinsic connectivity networks in the human brain to the presence of acoustic scanner noise. *NeuroImage, 55*, 1617–1632.

Larson, J. A. (1921). Modification of the Marson deception test. *Journal of Criminal Law and Criminology, 12*, 390–399.

Lashley, K. S. (1950). In search of the engram. *Symposia of the Society for Experimental Biology, 4*, 454–482.

Legrenzi, P., & Umiltà, C. A. (2011). *Neuromania: On the limits of brain science.* Oxford; New York: Oxford University Press.

Lehrer, J. (2010). The truth wears off: Is there something wrong with the scientific method? *The New Yorker.*

Lindquist, K. A., Wager, T. D., Kober, H., Bliss-Moreau, E., & Barrett, L. F. (2012). The brain basis of emotion. *Behavioral and Brain Sciences, 35*, 121–143.

Logothetis, N. K., Pauls, J., Augath, M., Trinath, T., & Oeltermann, A. (2001). Neurophysiological investigation of the basis of the fMRI signal. *Nature, 412*, 150–157.

Luce, R. D. (1959). *Individual choice behavior: A theoretical analysis.* New York: Wiley.

Luce, R. D. (1963). Detection and recognition. In R. D. Luce, R. R. Bush, & E. Galanter (Eds.), *Handbook of mathematical psychology* (Vol. 1, pp. 103–190). New York: Wiley.

Luce, R. D. (1977). Choice axiom after 20 years. *Journal of Mathematical Psychology, 15*(3), 215–233.

Luce, R. D., Bush, R. R., & Galanter, E. (1963). *Handbook of mathematical psychology,* Vol. 2. New York: Wiley.

Ludwig, K. (2003). The mind-body problem: An overview. In S. P. Stich & T. A. Warfield (Eds.), *The Blackwell guide to the philosophy of mind* (pp. 1–46). Malden, MA: Blackwell.

MacCorquodale, K., & Meehl, P. E. (1948). On a distinction between hypothetical constructs and intervening variables. *Psychological Review, 55*(2), 95–107.

Markram, H. (2006). The blue brain project. *Nature Reviews Neuroscience, 7*(2), 153–160.

Marks, W. B., Dobelle, W. H., & MacNichol, E. F.(1964). Visual pigments of single primate cones. *Science, 143*(361), 1181–1183.

Martin, S. J., Grimwood, P. D., & Morris, R.G.M. (2000). Synaptic plasticity and memory: An evaluation of the hypothesis. *Annual Review of Neuroscience, 23*, 649–711.

Mather, M., Cacioppo, J. T., & Kanwisher, N. (2013a). Introduction to the special section: 20 years of fMRI—What has it done for understanding cognition? *Perspectives on Psychological Science, 8*(1), 41–43.

Mather, M., Cacioppo, J. T., & Kanwisher, N. (2013b). How fMRI can inform cognitive theories. *Perspectives on Psychological Science, 8*(1), 108–113.

McCabe, D. P., & Castel, A. D. (2008). Seeing is believing: The effect of brain images on judgments of scientific reasoning. *Cognition, 107*(1), 343–352.

McClelland, J. L., & Rumelhart, D. E. (1986). *Parallel distributed processing: Explorations in the microstructure of cognition. Vol. 2: Psychological and biological models.* Cambridge, MA: MIT Press.

McGinn, C. (1989). Can we solve the mind body problem? *Mind, 98*(391), 349–366.

McGonigle, D. J., Howseman, A. M., Athwal, B. S., Friston, K. J., Frackowiak, R. S. J., & Holmes, A. P. (2000). Variability in fMRI: An examination of intersession differences. *NeuroImage, 11*(6), 708–734.

McIntosh, A. R. (2000). Towards a network theory of cognition. *Neural Networks, 13*(8–9), 861–870.

McMaster, R. (2011). Neuroeconomics: A sceptical view. *Real-World Economics Review, 58,* 113–125.

Meehl, P. E. (1978). Theoretical risks and tabular asterisks: Sir Karl, Sir Ronald, and the slow progress of soft psychology. *Journal of Consulting and Clinical Psychology, 46*(4), 806–834.

Mesulam, M. M. (1990). Large-scale neurocognitive networks and distributed-processing for attention, language, and memory. *Annals of Neurology, 28*(5), 597–613.

Miller, G. A. (2010). Mistreating psychology in the decades of the brain. *Perspectives on Psychological Science, 5*(6), 716–743.

Miller, M. B., Van Horn, J. D., Wolford, G. L., Handy, T. C., Valsangkar-Smyth, M., Inati, S., . . . Gazzaniga, M. S. (2002). Extensive individual differences in brain activations associated with episodic retrieval are reliable over time. *Journal of Cognitive Neuroscience, 14*(8), 1200–1214.

Modha, D. S., & Singh, R. (2010). Network architecture of the long-distance pathways in the macaque brain. *Proceedings of the National Academy of Sciences of the United States of America, 107*(30), 13485–13490.

Mole, C., & Klein, C. (2010). Confirmation, refutation, and the evidence of fMRI. In S. J. Hanson & M. Bunzl (Eds.), *Foundational issues in human brain mapping* (pp. 99–111). Cambridge, MA: MIT Press.

Moore, E. F. (1956). Gedanken-experiments on sequential machines. In C. E. Shannon & J. McCarthy (Eds.), *Automata studies* (pp. 129–156). Princeton, NJ: Princeton University Press.

Mukamel, R., Gelbard, H., Arieli, A., Hasson, U., Fried, I., & Malach, R. (2005). Coupling between neuronal firing, field potentials, and fMR1 in human auditory cortex. *Science, 309*(5736), 951–954.

Munk, H. (1881). *Uber die Funktionen der Grosshirnrinde.* Berlin: Hirschwald.

Nabavi, S., Fox, R., Proulx, C. D., Lin, J. Y., Tsien, R. Y., & Malinow, R. (2014). Engineering a memory with LTD and LTP. *Nature, 511*(7509), 348–352.

Nagel, E. (1979). *The structure of science: Problems in the logic of scientific explanation.* New York: Harcourt Brace and World.

Nemani, A. K., Atkinson, I. C., & Thulborn, K. R. (2009). Investigating the consistency of brain activation using individual trial analysis of high-resolution fMRI in the human primary visual cortex. *NeuroImage, 47*(4), 1417–1424.

Newton, I. (1687). *Philosophiæ naturalis principia mathematica.* Londini: Jussu Societatis Regiæ ac Typis Josephi Streater. Prostat apud plures Bibliopolas.

Nieuwenhuis, S., Forstmann, B. U., & Wagenmakers, E. J. (2011). Erroneous analyses of interactions in neuroscience: A problem of significance. *Nature Neuroscience, 14*(9), 1105–1107.

Nomura, E. M., Maddox, W. T., Filoteo, J. V., Ing, A. D., Gitelman, D. R., Parrish, T. B., . . . Reber, P. J. (2007). Neural correlates of rule-based and information–integration visual category learning. *Cerebral Cortex, 17*(1), 37–43.

Norman, K. A., Polyn, S. M., Detre, G. J., & Haxby, J. V. (2006). Beyond mind-reading: Multi-voxel pattern analysis of fMRI data. *Trends in Cognitive Sciences, 10*(9), 424–430.

Oosterwijk, S., Lindquist, K. A., Anderson, E., Dautoff, R., Moriguchi, Y., & Barrett, L. F. (2012). State of mind: Emotions, body feelings, and thoughts share distributed neural networks. *Neuroimage, 62,* 2110–2128.

Orban, G. A., Claeys, K., Nelissen, K., Smans, R., Sunaert, S., Todd, J. T., . . Vanduffel, W. (2006). Mapping the parietal cortex of human and non–human primates. *Neuropsychologia, 44*(13), 2647–2667.

Owen, A. M., Herrod, N. J., Menon, D. K., Clark, J. C., Downey, S. P., Carpenter, T. A., . . . Pickard, J. D. (1999). Redefining the functional organization of working memory processes within human lateral prefrontal cortex. [Research Support, Non-U.S. Gov't]. *European Journal of Neuroscience, 11*(2), 567–574.

Owen, A. M., McMillan, K. M., Laird, A. R., & Bullmore, E. (2005). N-back working memory paradigm: A meta-analysis of normative functional neuroimaging. *Human Brain Mapping, 25*(1), 46–59.

Page, M.P.A. (2006). What can't functional neuroimaging tell the cognitive psychologist? *Cortex, 42*(3), 428–443.

Palmer, S. E. (1999). *Vision science: Photons to phenomenology.* Cambridge, MA: MIT Press.

Papez, J. W. (1937). A proposed mechanism of emotion. *Archive of NeurPsych, 38,* 725–743.

Peelen, M. V., & Downing, P. E. (2005). Within-subject reproducibility of category-specific visual activation with functional MRI. *Human Brain Mapping, 25*(4), 402–408.

Peng, R. D. (2011). Reproducible research in computational science. *Science, 334*(6060), 1226–1227.

Place, U. T. (1956). Is consciousness a brain process? *British Journal of Psychology, 47*(1), 44–50.

Poldrack, R. A. (2006). Can cognitive processes be inferred from neuroimaging data? *Trends in Cognitive Sciences, 10*(2), 59–63.

Poldrack, R. A. (2008). The role of fMRI in Cognitive Neuroscience: where do we stand? *Current Opinion in Neurobiology, 18*(2), 223–226.

Poldrack, R. A. (2010). Mapping mental function to brain structure: How can cognitive neuroimaging succeed? *Perspectives on Psychological Science, 5*(6), 753–761.

Poldrack, R. A., Halchenko, Y., & Hanson, S. J. (2009). Decoding the large-scale brain structure classifying mental states across individuals. *Psychological Science, 20,* 1364–1372.

Poldrack, R. A., Mumford, J. A., & Nichols, T. E. (2011). *Handbook of Functional MRI data analysis.* Cambridge: Cambridge University Press.

Poline, J.-B., Thirion, B., Roche, A., & Meriaux, S. (2010). Intersubject variability in fMRI data: Causes, consequences and related analysis strategies. In S. J. Hanson & M. Bunzl (Eds.), *Foundational issues in human brain mapping* (pp. 173–191). Cambridge, MA: MIT Press.

Popper, K. (1963). *Conjectures and refutations.* London: Routledge and Kegan-Paul.

Posner, M. I., Petersen, S. E., Fox, P. T., & Raichle, M. E. (1988). Localization of cognitive operations in the human-brain. *Science, 240*(4859), 1627–1631.

Posner, M. I., & Rothbart, M. K. (2007). Research on attention networks as a model for the integration of psychological science. *Annual Review of Psychology, 58*, 1–23.

Posner, M. I., Sheese, B. E., Odludas, Y., & Tang, Y. Y. (2006). Analyzing and shaping human attentional networks. *Neural Networks, 19*(9), 1422–1429.

Powers, W. T. (2005). *Behavior: The control of perception.* New Canaan, CT: Benchmark Publications.

Price, C. J. (2010). The anatomy of language: a review of 100 fMRI studies published in 2009. *Year in Cognitive Neuroscience 2010, 1191*, 62–88.

Price, C. J., & Friston, K. J. (2005). Functional ontologies for cognition: The systematic definition of structure and function. *Cognitive Neuropsychology, 22*(3–4), 262–275.

Putnam, H. (1975). *Mind, language, and reality.* Cambridge; New York: Cambridge University Press.

Raichle, M. E., MacLeod, A. M., Snyder, A. Z., Powers, W. J., Gusnard, D. A., & Shulman, G. L. (2001). A default mode of brain function. *Proceedings of the National Academy of Sciences of the United States of America, 98*(2), 676–682.

Raichle, M. E., & Snyder, A. Z. (2007). A default mode of brain function: A brief history of an evolving idea [Commentary]. *NeuroImage, 37*, 1083–1090.

Rakover, S. S. (2011). A plea for a methodological dualism and a multi-explanation framework in psychology. *Behavior and Philosophy, 39*, 17–43.

Ramsey, J. D., Hanson, S. J., Hanson, C., Halchenko, Y. O., Poldrack, R. A., & Glymour, C. (2010). Six problems for causal inference from fMRI. [Research Support, Non-U.S. Gov't]. *NeuroImage, 49*(2), 1545–1558.

Redcay, E., & Courchesne, E. (2005). When is the brain enlarged in autism? A meta-analysis of all brain size reports. *Biological Psychiatry, 58*(1), 1–9.

Reid, A. T., Krumnack, A., Wanke, E., & Kotter, R. (2009). Optimization of cortical hierarchies with continuous scales and ranges. *NeuroImage, 47*(2), 611–617.

Roberts, S., & Pashler, H. (2000). How persuasive is a good fit? A comment on theory testing. *Psychological Review, 107*(2), 358–367.

Rumelhart, D. E., & McClelland, J. L. (1986). *Parallel distributed processing: Explorations in the microstructure of cognition. Vol. 1: Foundations.* Cambridge, MA: MIT Press.

Ryan, M. J. (2011). Replication in field biology: The case of the frog-eating bat. *Science, 334*(6060), 1229–1230.

Santer, B. D., Wigley, T.M.L., & Taylor, K. E. (2011). The reproducibility of observational estimates of surface and atmospheric temperature change. *Science, 334*(6060), 1232–1233.

Schooler, J. W., & Engstler-Schooler, T. Y. (1990). Verbal overshadowing of visual memories: Some things are better left unsaid. *Cognitive Psychology, 22*(1), 36–71.

Schroll, H., Vitay, J., & Hamker, F. H. (2012). Working memory and response selection: a computational account of interactions among cortico-basalganglio-thalamic loops. [Research Support, Non-U.S. Gov't]. *Neural Networks, 26*, 59–74.

Scoville, W. B., & Milner, B. (1957). Loss of recent memory after bilateral hippocampal lesions. *Journal of Neurology Neurosurgery and Psychiatry, 20*(1), 11–21.

Shinkareva, S. V., Mason, R. A., Malave, V. L., Wang, W., Mitchell, T. M., & Just, M. A. (2008). Using fMRI brain activation to identify cognitive states associated with perception of tools and dwellings. *PLOS One, 3*(1).

Simmonds, D. J., Pekar, J. J., & Mostofsky, S. H. (2008). Meta-analysis of Go/No-go tasks, demonstrating that fMRI activation associated with response inhibition is task-dependent. *Neuropsychologia, 46*(1), 224–232.

Simmons, J. P., Nelson, L. D., & Simonsohn, U. (2011). False-positive psychology: Undisclosed flexibility in data collection and analysis allows presenting anything as significant. *Psychological Science, 22*, 1359–1366.

Singh, I., & Rose, N. (2009). Biomarkers in psychiatry. *Nature, 460*(7252), 202–207.

Smith, A. J., Blumenfeld, H., Behar, K. L., Rothman, D. L., Shulman, R. G., & Hyder, F. (2002). Cerebral energetics and spiking frequency: The neurophysiological basis of fMRI. *Proceedings of the National Academy of Sciences of the United States of America, 99*(16), 10765–10770.

Smith, E. E., & Jonides, J. (1999). Neuroscience—Storage and executive processes in the frontal lobes. *Science, 283*(5408), 1657–1661.

Smith, S. M., Miller, K. L., Salimi-Khorshidi, G., Webster, M., Beckmann, C. F., Nichols, T. E., . . . Woolrich, M. W. (2011). Network modelling methods for FMRI. *NeuroImage, 54*(2), 875–891.

Sporns, O. (2011). *Networks of the brain*. Cambridge, MA: MIT Press.

Squire, L. R. (1992). Memory and the hippocampus: A synthesis from findings with rats, monkeys, and humans. *Psychological Review, 99*, 195–231.

Steele, J. M. (1974). Limit properties of Luce's choice theory. *Journal of Mathematical Psychology, 11*(2), 124–131.

Sternberg, S. (1969). Discovery of processing stages: Extensions of Donders' method. *Acta Psychologica, 30*, 276–315.

Sternberg, S. (2011). Modular processes in mind and brain. *Cognitive Neuropsychology, 28*(3–4), 156–208.

Stigler, S. M. (1986). *The history of statistics: The measurement of uncertainty before 1900*. Cambridge, MA: Belknap Press of Harvard University Press.

Tallis, R. (2011). *Aping mankind: Neuromania, Darwinitis, and the misrepresentation of humanity*. London: Acumen.

Thompson, R. F. (2005). In search of memory traces. *Annual Review of Psychology, 56*, 1–23.

Thyreau, B., Schwartz, Y., Thiriron, B., Frouin, V., Loth, E., Vollstädt-Klein, S . . . Poline, J.-B. (2012). Very large fMRI study using the IMAGEN database: Sensitivity-specificity and population effect modeling in relation to the underlying anatomy. *NeuroImage, 61*(1), 295–303.

Tomasello, M., & Call, J. (2011). Methodological challenges in the study of primate cognition. *Science, 334*(6060), 1227–1228.

Tomita, T. (1965). Electrophysiological study of mechanisms subserving color coding in fish retina. *Cold Spring Harbor Symposia on Quantitative Biology, 30*, 559–566.

Trepel, C., Fox, C. R., & Poldrack, R. A. (2005). Prospect theory on the brain? Toward a cognitive neuroscience of decision under risk. *Cognitive Brain Research, 23*(1), 34–50.

Tunturi, A. R. (1952). A difference in the representation of auditory signals for the left and right ears in the iso–frequency contours of the right middle ectosylvian auditory cortex of the dog. *American Journal of Physiology, 168*(3), 712–727.

Turkeltaub, P. E., Eden, G. F., Jones, K. M., & Zeffiro, T. A. (2002). Meta-analysis of the functional neuroanatomy of single-word reading: Method and validation. *NeuroImage, 16*(3), 765–780.

Uncapher, M. R., & Wagner, A.D. (2009). Posterior parietal cortex and episodic encoding: Insights from fMRI subsequent memory effects and dual-attention theory. *Neurobiology of Learning and Memory, 91*(2), 139–154.

Uttal, W. R. (1981). *A taxonomy of visual processes*. Hillsdale, NJ: L. Erlbaum Associates.

Uttal, W. R. (2001). *The new phrenology: The limits of localizing cognitive processes in the brain.* Cambridge, MA: MIT Press.

Uttal, W. R. (2005). *Neural theories of mind: Why the mind-brain problem may never be solved.* Mahwah, NJ: Lawrence Erlbaum Associates.

Uttal, W. R. (2011). *Mind and brain: A critical appraisal of cognitive neuroscience.* Cambridge, MA: MIT Press.

Uttal, W. R. (2012). *On the reliability of cognitive neuroscience data: A meta-meta-analysis.* Cambridge, MA: MIT Press.

Uttal, W. R. (2013). *Reliability in cognitive neuroscience: A meta-meta-analysis.* Cambridge, MA: MIT Press.

Vacariu, G., & Vacraiu, M. (2010). *Mind, life and matter in the hyperverse.* Bucharest: University of Bucharest Press.

Valenstein, E. S. (1998). *Blaming the brain.* New York: Free Press.

Van Essen, D. C., Anderson, C. H., & Felleman, D. J. (1992). Information processing in the primate visual system: An integrated systems perspective. *Science, 255*(5043), 419–423.

Van Orden, G. C., & Paap, K. R. (1997). Functional neuroimages fail to discover pieces of mind in parts of the brain. *Philosophy of Science Proceedings, 64,* S85–S94.

van Rooij, M., & Van Orden, G. (2011). It's about space, it's about time, neuroeconomics and the brain sublime. *Journal of Economic Perspectives, 25,* 31–56.

Vimal, R.L.P. (2009). Meanings attributed to the term 'consciousness': An overview. *Journal of Consciousness Studies, 16*(5), 9–27.

Vul, E., Harris, C., Winkielman, P., & Pashler, H. (2009). Puzzlingly high correlations in fMRI studies of emotion, personality, and social cognition. *Perspectives on Psychological Science, 4*(3), 274–290.

Vul, E., & Kanwisher, N. (2010). Begging the question: The nonindependence error in fMRI data analysis. In S. J. Hanson & S. M. Bunzi (Eds.), *Foundational issues for human brain mapping* (pp. 71–91). Cambridge, MA: MIT Press.

Wager, T. D., Jonides, J., & Reading, S. (2004). Neuroimaging studies of shifting attention: A meta-analysis. *NeuroImage, 22*(4), 1679–1693.

Wager, T. D., Phan, K. L., Liberzon, I., & Taylor, S. F. (2003). Valence, gender, and lateralization of functional brain anatomy in emotion: A meta-analysis of findings from neuroimaging. *NeuroImage, 19*(3), 513–531.

Wager, T. D., & Smith, E. E. (2003). Neuroimaging studies of working memory: A meta-analysis. *Cognitive, Affective, & Behavioral Neuroscience, 3*(4), 255–274.

Wang, J., Zuo, X., & He, Y. (2010). Graph-based network analysis of resting-state functional MRI. *Frontiers in Systems Neuroscience, 4,* 16.

Wastell, D., & White, S. (2012). Blinded by neuroscience: Social policy, the family, and the infant brain. *Families, Relationships, and Societies, 1,* 397–414.

Weisberg, D. S., Keil, F. C., Goodstein, J., Rawson, E., & Gray, J. R. (2008). The seductive allure of neuroscience explanations. *Journal of Cognitive Neuroscience, 20*(3), 470–477.

Wernicke, C. (1874). *Der aphasische Symptomencomplex.* Breslau: Teschen.

Winn, P. (2006). How best to consider the structure and function of the pedunculopontine tegmental nucleus: Evidence from animal studies. *Journal of the Neurological Sciences, 248*(1–2), 234–250.

Wittgenstein, L. (1958). *Preliminary studies for the "philosophical investigations," generally known as the blue and brown books.* Oxford: Blackwell.

Woolsey, C. N. (1952). *Pattern of localization in sensotry and motor areas of the cerebral cortex.* Paper presented at the The Biology of Mental Health and Disease: The Twentieth–seventh Annual Conference of the Millbank Memorial Fund, New York.

Yule, G. U. (1911). *An introduction to the theory of statistics.* London: C. Griffin and Company, limited.

Yule, G. U. (1926). Why do we sometimes get nonsense-correlations between time-series?—A study in sampling and the nature of time-series. *Journal of the Royal Statistical Society, 89*, 1–69.

INDEX